PERMANENT HEALING

includes quantum mechanics of healing

by

Daniel R. Condron
D.M., D.D., M.S.

SOM Publishing
Windyville, Missouri 65783

Other titles by Dr. Daniel R. Condron

- **Dreams of the Soul - The Yogi Sutras of Patanjali**
- **The Most Beautiful Book in the World**
- **Beyond Sales**
- **Beyond Phenomena - Readings from the Akasha**

Cover Art by David Varing
Cover Design and illustrations by Dave Lappin

ISBN: 0-944386-12-1

Library of Congress Catalogue Number pending

PRINTED IN THE UNITED STATES OF AMERICA

If you desire to learn more about the research and teachings in this book, write to School of Metaphysics, National Headquarters, Windyville, Missouri 65783. Or call 417-345-8411.

 The quality of your total health has a direct relationship with the quality of life you lead. This book is not intended to be used in lieu of professional health attention, rather it is a supplement of research and information to enhance ***Permanent Healing***. The author and publisher encourage the reader to seek second and third opinions concerning health disorders, as this is the right and choice of each individual in pursuing quality health care.

Something wonderful is happening.

A revolution is taking place.

This book is a mental revolution.

Your life is going to change.

Mankind will change.

What form will this change take?

This idea is so revolutionary it will answer the question, why?! Why did this happen to me? Why can't I ever have what I want? Why did my best friend or relative have to die?

These are questions people have asked them Selves throughout history. Very few have discovered the answer. Now, spelled out in black and white, for all to see and use are some of the solutions to the pain and misery suffered throughout and before recorded history.

These answers, ideas, and suggestions are given with love. They are given in the hope that they reach out to all who have a need and desire to heal them Selves, *PERMANENTLY*.

Contents

Foreword

To be asked to review, forward, or critique another writer's work is an honor, a compliment and a pleasurable responsibility.

I've known Dr. Daniel Condron as a neighbor, patient, fellow traveller on the Path, and a friend. Over the years, I watched the bloom of his spiritual awareness unfold as he patiently and with single-minded devotion sought and listened to the guidance of the Power within. I'm happy to see his progress which this work's coming into print represents.

There is a rhythmic law of life concerning reaping and sowing. This book is an expression of the sowing so those who follow might reap.

I can't remember when I didn't want to be a doctor, a healer. My mother was a nurse, and as a weak and sickly child, I had the opportunity to benefit continuously from her caring efforts. When she would be ill, it was I who was inclined to try to care for her. My poor health kept the healer dream at bay until age 17. An aunt directed my parents to Dr. Puls, a chiropractor in Miamisburg, Ohio, who began turning my health status around. Soon I knew I could realize my goal and wanted to be his kind of doctor.

Little did I know then my foot had just been placed on the route which would wind through so many varied avenues of experience which, if written, would be more easily accepted as "fiction rather than fact" for leaping the barricades "protecting" each of us, until evolutionarily ready, from the growth on the inner realms is not easy nor can it be forced upon ourselves or upon others.

Can one see both sides of a coin simultaneously? Can one breathe in and out at the same time? Can one eat the beautifully decorated cake without cutting it? Can one serve both God and mammon, as a famous book references? It seems an either/or world, doesn't it?

However, the "yes" answers to such questions revealed themselves as I gradually left the either/or concept and became more and more an and/also person. I never was good at puzzles or riddles, and still miss the answers to them when relying on my "educated mind" as Dr. Palmer referenced it. Magicians can always fool me right in front of my eyes. We all first live in fantasy and then find growing up involves giving it up. Wisdom later returns it to us as a useful tool to enjoy, for Truth is there as everywhere.

When I enrolled as a freshman in chiropractic college, I had no idea the next few years would find me in the dangerous storm of establishing a new profession legally and socially. I went from a minor practice to the top two percent of the profession in income and traffic. I had a large practice, seeing 150 to 185 patients per day. We doctors were arrested and tried in court, suffered great personal sacrifices, threats to our lives, experienced the organized power and cunning and hatred of the established "They" and felt the danger and loneliness of walking an unlighted tightrope, maintaining balance and progress only because of an unseen spiritual nudge.

It wasn't until my health broke down from the strain of all this and death was about to ring the doorbell that a barrier to my door of consciousness was cracked. From then on a period filled with rapid growth of the inner faculties, phenomena beyond my immediate comprehension, and a view ahead and behind in time connected my life with both purpose and direction.

Healing patients' bodies, as remarkable as so many of the experiences were, was good, but there always seemed to be something more needed. I entered a course of study, (I learned what was meant by Magnificent Obsession), and at one point felt I'd finally realized my goal of working with the complete person - body, mind, soul.

For patients to realize the connection between his or her emotions and attitudes is a major step toward changing, for the better, their patterns of illness and reaching permanent healing. We are all constantly in a stage of becoming. The only static thing in life is change. We could have asked above, "Can something be still and moving at the same time?"

Everyone is seeking whether aware of it or not. Fortunate are you who will be reading this to know you are a seeker. Seek on and reap. More Love and Light to you.

——David C. McKnight, D.C.

PERMANENT HEALING
Section I

Introduction

At a very early age I discovered the power of my thoughts. My early childhood was a continual battle with illness. Each week I was given a shot by the doctor at the hospital. I was given pills. I experienced times of dizziness and times when my body would "freeze" into an almost paralyzed state.

Two weeks before my seventh birthday, while sitting in the waiting room of our family doctor's office with my mother, I found myself unable to catch my breath. I was rushed into the doctor's office where I was given a injection which aided my breathing. I was then taken to the hospital and placed in an oxygen tent where I remained overnight. That night I endured many more shots. This was not a very pleasant day for a seven year old. This episode was preceeded by two weeks of sickness and absence from school.

The next day, my parents took me home. I recovered. I turned seven years old a couple of weeks later. After my seventh birthday I never had a problem with my breathing again. In fact, I was one of the healthiest children throughout the rest of grade school and high school. As a senior, I was captain of my high school basketball team, all conference, three sport letterman and still found time to serve as president of the student body of my school.

What caused this miraculous turn-around? The power of thought. A child, up to the age of seven, is like a sponge in that they absorb information from the environment. This is not only information received through the five senses, but also the emotions, thoughts, and attitudes of those in the environment.

By the age of seven, the child has enough data in the brain to begin the process of reasoning. The child begins to think for himself and to exert his own free will more and more.

This is exactly what occurred with me. By the age of seven, I was forming many of my own conclusions. I had begun the process of correlating an experience stored in my brain's memory with an event I was currently experiencing. At other times I would perceive a relationship between two events separated by time. These two events were both being stored in my brain as memory.

This ability to choose my own thoughts created a freedom in my thinking and therefore in my life. This freedom from restriction in thinking processes produced a freedom from restriction in my ability to breathe easily.

I was able to think my way to health, as well as success in life. The steps I used then, as well as the many steps I have discovered and used over the past thirty years, are the subject of this book. You will find this to be a sourcebook for thought and attitude difficulties which create physical disorder, dis-ease, and illness. Even more importantly, you will find within these pages the answer to the question "Why did this happen to me?" You will find the mental attitude cause of your physical disorder. I have also provided mental and physical steps that may be applied to give the user a method to develop the new, more productive thought form and attitude.

I am happy and excited to be able to give this information and experience to the world for it has the potential to aid in not only relieving pain and suffering but to lift mankind to a new level of awareness of the power of thought. With this knowledge and awareness we can create a better world.

Rev. Dr. Daniel R. Condron

Puppies

My family always had dogs on our farm. At least once a year one of the females would give birth to a litter of puppies. I found much joy in playing with these puppies and taking care of them. I would feed them and as they got older would take them with me on walks through the woods. I would usually choose my favorite pup from the litter and give the pup a name. This one I would give extra attention. My brothers and sisters would choose their favorite also.

I noticed over the years, the puppy I chose and gave extra attention to grew up to have a personality distinct from the others.

I began to experiment. I would choose two pups from a litter and give a name to each one. Then I would treat each one differently. I would always smile and have a happy voice while playing with one puppy. The other I would raise with a strict voice, being very firm and serious about anything I was doing or saying with this dog.

The result was that by the time of maturity, the first dog was happy-go-lucky, always smiling, very energetic. The second dog did not smile nearly as much, looked down a lot, didn't wag its tail much but did crave attention. Animals habitually adopt thoughts and attitudes of their owner, trainer, or other people in their environment.

People also are raised in a variety of ways, by all kinds of parents with varying personalities. We are raised according to our parents' limitations, including their exceptional traits and their weaknesses. Many people accept the limitations their parents have taught them and teach the same unproductive attitudes to their children. These unproductive or negative attitudes over time produce in the grown up children similar physical dis-ease, disorder and illness.

Therefore, you will find a family member saying, "Well, my mother had arthritis and that is why I have it," or "my father always had hay fever so I guess I inherited the hay fever from him."

It isn't the physical inheritance that is a factor in many parent-child similar disorders. It is the mental inheritance, for you have inherited your parents' mental attitudes. Some of these thought patterns may be very valuable, whereas others may keep you in a state of pain and dissatisfaction.

A habitual person, an individual with a weak will who accepts the limitations of others as his own, will stop growing at about the age of 18 and will remain mentally similar to his parents for the rest of his life.

The determined individual with clearly imagined goals will appreciate everything productive his parents and teachers taught him exhibiting the highest respect for his teachers by going beyond his parent's limitations, creating on a larger, more expansive scale.

If a parent accepted resentment in his life, his strong offspring will replace it with creating purpose for everything he does. If a parent practiced and taught guilt and condemnation, the determined offspring will replace it with seeing the beauty of the now, present experience and imagine new, more expansive goals for the Self.

No matter what environment you were raised in, poor or wealthy, restrictive or expansive, you have the capability to rise above those limitations. This process begins by examining your attitudes and replacing the unproductive with productive ones. The specific attitudes, their physical results on the body and suggestions for correction and improvement, are given in this book.

Concerning Death

How many times have you gone to a funeral and asked your Self, "Why did such a wonderful person have to die at such a young age?" Perhaps, the person was older, and you still wondered why they had to leave you.

Most untimely deaths could have been prevented. It is each individual's right to decide if they are going to be sick or well. We do owe it to each person to aid them to move out of non-awareness of the causal factors of illness. In this way should they decide to become well and whole, they will have the tools at their disposal to do so.

Sometimes cancer kills, sometimes it doesn't. Many people have hepatitis and it doesn't kill them. Why do some people contract an illness and it kills them, while others come down with the same illness, recover and live for many years?

Now, with this revolutionary book, people can <u>know</u> why they are dying. Also friends and relatives can know, not just <u>believe</u> , why a loved one is dying. Consequently, you achieve peace of mind. You <u>know</u> the cause and can do your best to aid the individual.

Life is meant to be one vast learning opportunity. Restrictive attitudes will over time reduce the learning both in quality and in quantity of time allowed for maturing. Gaining a knowledge of the mind and its mental effect on the body will give control to any person willing to invest a little time and energy into Self growth and Self improvement.

Another benefit of knowing the attitudes that cause physical illness is awareness of the thinking process of world leaders. Anytime you read a newspaper and find out a world leader is ill then you can discern the restrictive thinking creating this illness. When the president of this country comes down with the common cold you realize he is being indecisive and needs to make a decision. An awareness of the causal factors behind world events proceeding from world leaders can be a source of great satisfaction as well as giving the inside track on investments.

Recognize that health is a state of mind and more importantly it is a specific state of mind. Death occurs when the thought-attitude-thinking becomes so restrictive that learning no longer occurs. Now there is hope, for this book brings the evolutionary educational process for the Self recovery of a more expansive and abundant life.

Authority

All creation begins with a mental construct, a thought picture. We have created our physical bodies the way they are today with our thoughts and attitudes. Knowing this, you can gain a great deal more confidence for if you had the power to create illness or disease, you also have the power to create wholeness and a state of health.

Authority and control of your life always begins with having a clear mental picture of who you want to be and how you want your life to be. Many times I am asked by individuals if they should stay in a relationship. I tell them that is their decision to make but they do need to have a clear mental image of what qualities they desire in a relationship. Then they can begin to discern the degree to which they have manifested their ideal association.

When you have a clear, detailed, mental image of what is desired in life or in a specific area of your life, the process of building and understanding authority has already begun. In every word you speak you will be describing the plan. Every action will move you closer to the desired outcome. Others may marvel at your directedness and your ability to stay on track. You will be able to speak as someone who knows what he is talking about for, in fact, you *will* know. Action directed toward this clear mental image will produce fulfilling results.

This same process will work very well for changing disorders to health in your physical body. Not only must you imagine your physical body to be the way you desire but also by knowing the attitude producing the disorder you will change that mental picture.

No longer will you feel out of control when your body isn't functioning correctly, for you will be aware of the Self created cause and you have the power to change it! You can change resentment to a purposeful life, fear to desire, weakness to power, and low Self worth to value. You will have authority.

Love

I honestly believe and have come to know that love is more powerful than hate. I have seen sharing and teaching given with love continue on and on. I have seen seemingly powerful individuals who fell victim to hate, destroy themselves and much of their environment.

Love lasts. Love sustains. Love gives, and gives and gives. In the end love always receives. In the uninhibited giving through the laws of the universe, time, effort, and energy given freely with the best of intentions will return in abundance to the giver.

Never forget this: what you give freely, with the best of intentions, with love, will return to you and you will prosper both in health and wealth as well as friendship.

What is a friend? How do you recognize a true friend? How shall a true friend be known? How can you be certain when true friendship exists? The answer is this. A friend is a person who aids or helps you fulfill inner desires. This does not mean accumulating all the possessions in the world. This does entail aiding another person along the road of life and helping them in their learning and growth. It means teaching and giving to others the valuable lessons of life you have discovered and found to be true. For truly, as you help others to lead a happier, healthier existence, you help yourself to the same. You, the giver, the teacher, however, now reach a higher level of learning and existence for there is truth to the old adage, he who teaches learns.

As you learn to give and teach and pass on what you are learning, you gradually become a world server, a world class teacher.

This is a teacher of the highest order for you are teaching the Master Subject: Mind, Self and uplifting of humanity.

True love for all humanity is experienced when we create avenues to give to all humanity. Through giving and teaching, the state of awareness on the whole planet is improved and progression towards enlightenment occurs.

Begin each day by loving your Self. End each day by loving your Self. Share your love and giving in between, all day long. You will find your world opens to you and your capacity to receive increases 10-fold, over and over.

Love to give by recognizing that what you give forth freely will return freely with interest. The energy of the universe is never wasted. Nothing is ever wasted by nature. Therefore, do not waste your time, energy, thoughts, money, or health by hoarding. Rather, give freely of your time and attention to the individuals of the universe and it will return to you in abundance.

This is the most important point to keep in mind and practice in order to overcome the disorders mentioned in this book. There are specific mental causes for the physical disorders given. Recognize and be aware of your intention at all times. Make sure it is a productive intention and live life to the fullest.

Communication for Healing

Once a person has experienced or suffered mental, emotional, or physical pain, the result is trauma. Some people carry this trauma with them for the rest of their life allowing it to interfere with the correct and accurate perception of people, places, objects, and experiences in the present.

This attachment to trauma inhibits learning for the individual continues to relive the past through memory which clouds the present day experiences. In order to release this trauma or pain, it must be brought to the surface where it can be examined in the light of awareness. The trauma must be discussed for the first step to permanent healing is communication.

As you describe the source of pain, the mental and emotional hurts are identified more specifically. Eventually, the cause is perceived and correction begins. A mental attitude was begun by your Self and formed over time. Therefore, it will require time and effort to adjust the thinking to a more productive mode. The length of time will be determined by the amount of effort expended in correction. The correction will however be worth every bit of effort many times over.

We often hide behind words. We use them or misuse them as a facade to hide our true thoughts.

I have known many people who have used the word *perfect* as a way of punishing themselves. They have been taught since childhood that they are supposed to be *perfect*. Yet, they are not perfect. Therefore, these people must condemn themselves, hurt themselves and be angry with themselves, in their own mind. In short, they think they are bad because they are not perfect. Let's take a look at the word *perfect*. If you are perfect, how could you change? For if you are perfect there is nothing more to do or to learn which is nothing more than stagnancy or non-change or non-growth. Without growth there is no life. Death occurs when there is no learning or no growth.

So instead of striving for perfection and punishing Self when you are less than perfect, place the attention on adding to the productive qualities and value you already have. No one can ever be perfect for our universe is one of continual change and motion. Identify with forward motion and growth and you will lead a happy and satisfying life.

The Body is a Feedback System for the Mind

As amazing as it seems the mind has provided for our needs. Whenever one can ask a question, there is an answer. A question most everyone has asked sometime in their life is, "Why did this happen to me?" This question usually follows a traumatic experience. One of the most devastating experiences we can encounter is that of ill health. Suddenly we find ourselves to one degree or another immobile. Even the common cold can be a very bothersome experience.

To get about fulfilling the duties and joys of life, we need a healthy, well functioning body-vehicle. If we want to walk a distance we need feet, legs, hips and lungs that function efficiently. When we eat, we need to have a mouth, throat, teeth, tongue, stomach, and intestines that work efficiently. When we use a typewriter, we expect our eyesight, hearing, sense of touch and coordination to serve us well. When we lift an object, we expect to have strong muscles, back vertebrae in good shape and in alignment, with joints and ligaments in working order.

The body is such an advanced, elaborate, and specific feedback mechanism that it provides clues and answers even to mental and emotional pain and anguish. The body is so <u>specific</u> in its language that it lets any person know the exact mental attitude that is holding back their progression and causing the pain.

For example, the common cold may be used to inform one of the need to make a decision and stop doubting one's own ability. Kidney stones and difficulty in the urinary system point to the need to stop living in the failures of the past and the need to concentrate on creating success in the present. Difficulties with the liver signal a need to start respecting yourself and create a purpose for living. Difficulties in the area of the pancreas signal the need to give more of yourself in time, energy, and friendship to others. The question has been asked, "If what you say is true, that we do in fact cause our own physical illnesses or dis-ease through the action of our attitudes then does this mean I am a bad or terrible person? After all, why would I do such a terrible thing to myself?" The answer is: need for awareness, lack of education, or ignorance concerning this area of knowledge. In the years to come this knowledge will become available to the entire world and there will be general awareness concerning it.

The major point to realize is that no matter where you are concerning your physical health, there can be a possibility of improvement. Some, upon reading the mental attitude that causes the physical disorder will say, "but I am not like that." My suggestion to those people is to practice watching their thoughts for one week. Write down and keep a list of every negative thought you have during that week. Write about each anger, fear, doubt, worry, guilt, condemnation, jealousy or manipulation thought you experience. List every *I can't, I shouldn't, I won't, I haven't*. In short, list all the *not's*, all the negations, all the limitations placed on Self by Self for one week.

At the end of the week you will begin to perceive your mental restrictions and have enough data to begin to isolate the area of restriction for your Self. This is the attitude disorder causing illness.

Permanent Healing

This book would not be complete without a discussion of those unconscious factors that figure into an individual's personality.

We have received training from our parents and environment through our early years, but we have not looked to see why certain factors occur.

There is an old story told of the mother who always cut off the end of her roast before she placed it in the oven. Her daughter learned from her mother to cut the end of the roast off before cooking. The daughter then taught this roast-cutting to her daughter. One day the daughter's daughter's husband asked her, "Why do you always cut off the ends of your roast?" She said, "Well, that is the way my mother always did it." So then she went to her mother and asked her the same question to which her mother replied, "Well, I don't know, because that is the way my mother always cooked roast." So then the daughter and mother went to the grandmother and asked, "Why do you always cut the ends off your roast beef before you put it in the oven?" The answer from the grandmother was, "Because the whole time you were growing up I always had a small roasting pan and the roast would not fit in the pan unless I cut the ends off."

The answer is they were performing this habitual behavior of cooking roast without understanding the reason or purpose for it. The average person operates this way to one degree or another most of the time.

Imagine this one instance, then reflect back on 18 years of infancy, adolescence, and striving towards adulthood before you moved out on your own. All this time you were being influenced and trained in limited ways of thinking by parents and, to a lesser degree, others in your environment. You begin to see the tremendous effect your physical family had on your ways of thinking whether or not you choose to think that way consciously, reasoningly, and willfully. Then include your schooling, your church, organizations, community, and you can also see the tremendous influence on the way you lead your life, act and react now as an adult. You are in many ways formed by the way you are trained by those around you, consciously or unconsciously on their part. This training is habitual or willful to the degree of their limitations and awareness.

When we begin the study of the Self, we begin to recognize those factors that are not reasonable or sensible anymore. There are certain reactions that cause specific unpleasantness in our lives.

We begin to ask our Selves, "Would a different way cause greater learning and growth? Would I be happier and enjoy my life? Would my life be more satisfying and fulfilling? Would I grow and learn and change and add to myself, evolving more?" These are important questions to ask. We are continually reacting to what someone says or the way a person acts or a certain type of person. We just can't stand the way they say things.

You begin to think about this and say to your Self, "Why do I react to this? Why do I get embarrassed about certain situations and no one else does? Why do I get angry in certain situations and no one else does?"

These angers, resentments, guilts, fears, doubts, and worries will point us to areas where there is a desire to gain further and greater learning about ourselves.

As you are reading through this compilation, this glossary of attitudes and disease/illnesses, you will see the physical illness and then the mental disorder. An emotional reaction to your environment is also an indication of dis-ease or a dis-order that will point the way to the desire or need to learn. In many of these cases, you will read in the glossary about an attitude and then in my suggestions I will say this comes from a fear or doubt or limitation. When you see this, you will begin to recognize your own reactions and the way they become apparent. For example, Self hate is the cause of cancer. Many times this hate is directed outward to the environment as a hatred for someone else or to many people in the environment. When the hatred becomes very strong it develops into a hatred for almost everyone. Perhaps, you see the whole world as your enemy.

Self condemnation is the attitude that is a factor in bringing about kidney stones in the body. You may remember a time when you felt guilt or remorse for something you said to someone. Your condemnation was the indication of an attitude needing to be changed. Instead of mentally beating your Self, you create compassion and love for healing to occur.

These types of reactions are our clues. They indicate areas where we lack Self control. When we have reactions, it is important to look at why we have them, where we formulated them, why we carry them around with us, and what we need to do to change them into a more productive way of thinking and living.

At this point look over the different attitudes and dis-eases/ illnesses. Be aware of people in your environment. Look for other examples demonstrating how most people are unconscious of their own reactions and the way they react to everyday situations. You will notice that many times people don't have enough attention on their thoughts to see the source of their reactions or how they can change them.

Cause Always Begins with a Thought, Everything Else is Sub-Cause

I enjoy reading and learning about various areas of the field of health and healing. I also enjoy talking to people in these areas because each experience is an education.

Today, there are many different fields that anyone can investigate in order to learn about the wholistic approach to healing. Since each individual is unique, their needs are also unique. Various fields may provide relief to some, while others may benefit more from another field of healing. Naturopathy, naprapathy, herbology, acupressure, acupuncture, foot reflexology, nutrition, and homeopathy are all areas that attempt to aid the person to find relief so he can lead a more productive life.

I also love history. In high school, history was my favorite subject. I enjoy reading about the history of chiropractic. I enjoy reading the history of osteopathy. Although I am not a homeopath, I enjoy reading about and discovering more of the history of homeopathy. It seems that during the latter half of the nineteenth century and the early part of the 20th century, homeopathy was a very predominate area of the health and healing field. At that time over one-fourth of all practicing doctors were homeopaths. In fact, there were even homeopathic hospitals.

History is full of examples and in many ways is a record of the efforts people have made to improve their way of life. The field of healing is no exception to this. Chiropractic was founded because a person discovered a way to relieve people's suffering and aid them to better health. Acupuncture, although it has existed and been used productively in China for many thousand of years, is now available in the West because it offers relief from suffering in ways that some individuals had not been able to find before. Herbs had been used since ancient times for man's well-being. Civilized man had until recently forgotten about the beneficial effects of these. I appreciate and applaud these individuals who are making this knowledge available to the common man. Naprapathy was developed from a person's desire to improve the ability to aid others by treating not only the bones, but also the ligaments, tendons and muscles.

Thoughts have reality. Therefore, your thoughts affect your whole life and the physical reality around you, not just your physical body environment but your outward environment too. Fortunately, for most people, the manifestation of their thoughts is not instantaneous. Thoughts require lag time to become a part of our physical lives. There is usually a delay between the time you think a thought and the time it occurs in your life. This delay time affords you time to prepare your Self for the repercussions of your thoughts. Ask your Self, "What was I thinking about ten minutes ago, ten hours ago, and ten days ago?" If you cannot answer these questions, then you will have difficulty understanding why situations, circumstances, and events occur in your life. You will constantly be asking your Self, "Why did this happen to me?"

When you have a thought or attitude, it becomes stronger and stronger as you think about it. If you think thoughts of hate, those thoughts will become stronger each time you dwell on hate. Eventually, the thought will become so strong that it affects your emotions. You will become emotionally irritable. You may react with anger or Self pity easily. Gradually, the anger or related emotion will become so strong that your emotions can no longer contain it. It then must move out into your physical body as illness or disease. From here, it may affect your whole life reducing your productivity, driving away friends and costing you your job.

The physical body is the second line of resistance to unproductive thoughts. The first line of resistance is your emotions. The third line of defense is those around you. All fields and studies of healing fall under this category of treating these lines of resistance or defense. The closer they get and the farther they go to treating first cause, which is thought, the more directly they effect permanent healing.

How can we aid the body to repair itself? The speed or quickness of repair depends on what has been learned concerning the causal factor of the illness. In order to have a healing that is lasting we need to treat both the specific illness and the whole system. The specific illness gives us the first indication, like a meter reading, of what is occurring both with the physical body and mental attitudes.

For example, suppose you are preparing to drive a car. You look at the speedometer noticing it reads 0 miles per hour. The speedometer gives an indication of the speed of movement of the car. Now, imagine you have your foot on the accelerator, you press down and the car goes forward. So you say, "Eureka! I have discovered the cause of the car moving forward."

One day you find that acceleration is very sluggish when you press the accelerator with your foot. Upon further investigation it is discovered that the spark plugs are corroded and need to be replaced. Accomplishing this, you find the car accelerates very well. Now you say, "I have found the cause of my car going slow! I understand how to fix it and make it run fast so I know the cause of a car running fast is good spark plugs."

Until one day you have problems with the transmission. You engage the transmission, putting the car into gear, and you hear a sound that goes clank-clank-clank. Something drops on the ground and you can't go anywhere. So you say to yourself, "Maybe I ought to get this fixed." You take the car to somebody who knows how to fix transmissions. You help them to fix the transmission in order to save yourself some money. In the process you learn all about transmissions. Your transmission is fixed and the car runs smoother than it ever did before. You say to yourself, "Now I know the reason why my car moves so fast because I see the connection between the motor and transmission. They work together to cause the tires to move and propel the car. Now I understand why the car goes forward."

I could go on and on with examples of your personal discovery of why a car moves forward. What is the cause? Which one of these is the cause and reason for the car traveling at high speed?

Is the driver the cause? You can go into a junk yard and sit in a car. Put your foot on the accelerator and see if you travel at 55 m.p.h. Are you the cause in this case? Are you the cause of driving a working, functioning car? Does the driver determine how fast the car will travel? If this is so will your car travel at 250 miles per hour? Only if you possess a car that will travel that rate of speed. So you see there are a lot of different ramifications with this idea of "cause". If we wanted to search for original cause, we might research the early pioneers of the automobile industry. We could discover that before the automobile was developed, the bicycle with a chain drive was invented. The older type of bicycle with the front wheel larger than the back wheel was more like a two wheeled version of our modern day tricycle. The earliest cars used the technology that preceded them. So instead of a transmission, these earliest cars used a chain drive like the bicycles that preceded them. In fact, the earliest cars looked like buggies without horses. They were referred to as horseless carriages. Instead of being propelled by a horse, they utilized the internal combustion engine. Nowadays we refer to the power an engine develops as *horsepower* which is the unit of measurement for that power. The factors that lead to the development of the automobile began before the horse and buggy, the bicycle, and many other inventions.

Your physical body is not a car, yet, it does have many working parts. In order for you to experience health, all these parts must be in working order and functioning in harmony with the whole system. Just as the modern automobile is the result of over one hundred years of evolution and contains thousands of parts working together, so the human body is a product of millions of years of evolution and product development. To perform efficiently, the body and its constituent parts need to be in peak working order.

There were hundreds and perhaps thousands of inventions developed before an internal combustion engine could be developed to propel the automobile. Why is a book on permanent healing presenting the history of the automobile? The answer is a car is a vehicle that you use to move your physical body from one locale to another while the physical body is a vehicle the soul or inner Self uses to move from one locale to another for experiencing, learning, and growth in our physical life.

There is a cause for you, the thinker, having a physical body. Evolution is this process of development. We read the records the anthropologists discover concerning the bones and fossils of ancient man and the records the biologists present of DNA and the genetic code. We trace the evolution of man's physical body back through earlier ancestors called homo sapiens, Neanderthal, homo habilus, homo erectus and others. We continue to discover that the evolution of the physical body as we use it today has been in the process of developing for many millions of years.

So it is with the automobile. The similarity is the automobile for the past one hundred years has been undergoing a process of evolution and development to meet the needs of a developing humanity. You can abuse or mistreat your car as you can refuse to take care of your physical body. You neglect your body if you don't get enough food, water, shelter, clothing, or sleep. If you don't eat enough food, after a while you won't have the energy to be able to function on your job or other activities you desire. You won't have enough calories which is a unit of measure of energy. If you refuse to drink water or some type of liquid then in a very short time your body will not be able to perform for you, the thinker.

In looking to discover the mental cause of physical illness or dis-ease, look at the thoughts a person has about their physical body and taking care of it. Now suppose you are given a car for the first time. You don't know anything about it, but you are given a car and something breaks down. You don't know what it is. You call somebody to fix it and, believe it or not, this is the way most people are. They don't know much about their physical body so when it breaks down, they call somebody to fix it. They contact someone who will cut or sew or give a shot or just say, "Eat chicken soup and stay in bed for three days." But, if we know when the body breaks down what specific area is the difficulty, then we can find what the cause of the difficulty is.

My investigations show that cause always proceeds from a mental attitude. For example, you might say, "Well, I've got a cold because it is cold season and everybody else's cold got around and I've caught it from somebody." This is very true. It seems to make all the sense in the world, doesn't it? An outside virus carried by someone else is the cause of your current malady. But just like the car, pushing on the accelerator, it seems like the cause, but there is a deeper cause. You need to look at the engine.

Why is it that Joe, your best friend, two desks apart from you at the office didn't get a cold and you did? Why is it that everyone in the office got a cold but you didn't? If a cold is a virus doesn't it seem like you should be able to withstand a virus if you are in proper mental condition? After all, mankind has spent millions of years developing this body to be able to withstand viruses.

Did you know that if your immunological system didn't function, you probably wouldn't live twenty-four hours? So there seems to be a cause, an attitude, that relates to the defense system breaking down.

As another example, let's say you have a pain in your back and you desire to get the misaligned vertebra in place. So you say to yourself, "Okay, the misaligned vertebra is the cause of my pain. I'll get my bones adjusted." Again you are correct in your statement. The last time I went to a chiropractor, he put some needles in me and then, at the end, he adjusted my neck, never touching my back or spine. He said, "Well, I could adjust the other parts but the needles work with the energy to balance your system."

So evidently there are causes other than those we have heretofore examined. There is a reason for vertebrae to shift out of place, out of alignment. We can look to discover what these causes are. In a like manner, we might look to discover the cause of a weakened organ in the body. We could look to see what attitudes would cause disorder in the kidneys. Now consider, if you've earned the right as man to be a thinker, you must have earned the right to choose the thoughts you have, productive or unproductive, especially since we all seem to have free will. If you can choose thought and if you can cause your mind to be productive, doesn't it make sense that you, driver of your vehicle (body), is capable of causing productivity in that body?

This is the basic premise of this book: *thoughts have power, thoughts are real, and you create your physical body each day by the thoughts and attitudes you create and maintain.* Attitudes are particular thought patterns repeated over a period of time.

As one progresses and grows, the individuality is improved and enhanced. Each of us becomes a greater creator in our own right and in our separate creations we form a truly unique individuality. As we progress and grow, we gain in uniqueness and diversity. Our differences are seen to be only temporary steps to understanding our common goal of wisdom and enlightenment.

Each of us holds two abilities that were gifts when we were created. These are free will and individuality. Each one of us is an individual. You can recognize this individuality in the physical body because we are not connected at the head. We are individuals. You make decisions each day that have nothing to do with me. We are individuals and we have free will. You make decisions that are personally your decisions. If everyone on this planet came one step away from spiritual maturity, would we all look the same? The answer is no. The answer is no because we would all have super-powerful creative thought forms and our body would respond to these powerful thought forms. Since we would determine our physical body, this would include our looks or appearance.

A woman I knew said she was having some problems and it had begun to affect her physically. She knew her body didn't feel quite right so she sat down and started writing. She wrote 18 pages of hand-written material which was something she normally did not do. She said she felt such a relief afterwards. Next she went into the bathroom to wash her face and looked at herself in the mirror. She said, "You know, I looked at myself and I actually looked pretty." I had never thought of her as being anything other than pretty before but evidently she had and the important point is that she noticed a dramatic physical difference in her face. My response was, "Well, that makes all the sense in the world because your face will show your identity. Your face represents your identity. If you release the pressure you are holding inside yourself, your face is going to relax. The muscles in your face will relax instead of holding tension and there is going to be a prettier look immediately." A change in attitude can bring about a very rapid change in the body. The color of your eyes also can change depending on your thoughts.

I have been asked if I think we will ever get to the point in our evolutionary development where we will lose our individuality. My answer is no. In fact quite the opposite is true. The further we progress on the evolutionary or spiritual ladder of self development, the greater awareness and understanding we have of ourselves as individual creators. Individuality is maximized as we grow. We find the greatest fulfillment in our individuality as we are creators. We have the most to offer others who are learning and developing their understanding of Self as creator. Would we all think the same and look the same? It would never happen. The more creative you are, the more you advance as a creator, the more you evolve, the less boring you are and the more exciting you are.

If you have gaps in your learning there will be a tendency to repeat the same mistakes. Why? Because you don't have memory of the past. Even more important, most everyone has experienced making the same mistake more than once. You knew better, or you saw it when it came up twice, saying, "I should have changed back then, but I didn't, and now I'm going to change."

Donna always seemed to have problems. She was always either getting beaten or beating someone else. This beating usually was emotional, mental, or verbal, but sometimes physical as well. The effect on her body was staggering. She had heart problems, gall bladder problems, cranial and spinal problems, and other physical disorders. I observed her receiving physical treatments and in a matter of hours the symptoms would return because her attitudes remained the same.

When life hits you in the face or you get knocked down a few times, you can change for the better. Another example is finding out about a success story and being aware of the factors that caused that success yet failing to use what is known when the opportunity presents itself. Much later, after many pains and troubles, you decide it is worth the effort to practice and repeat the success.

Another question I have been asked is why would anyone choose to be born into a deformed body. For example, why would a soul choose a deformed brain providing very little capabilities for reasoning? In that situation, there couldn't be a great deal added to the Self without the reasoning factor, but there could occur a balancing process. The balancing occurs in giving freely because we know as you give, so shall you receive. In order for learning to occur there must be giving present. Imagine putting yourself in a situation where there would be just one or two ways that you would be able to give.

Consider, if you were existing in a physical body that was so restricted you could only give to others in one or two ways. One of these ways would be love. Your body would not function properly so there would be a need to be taken care of by others. Suppose you are a very loving child, but the physical body does not function well. In this condition, the child would have the opportunity to give unconditional love. There would be few distractions from giving so it would be focused on one specific area. You might have the opportunity to practice receiving also because people would be taking care of you most of the time.

You are here in the physical environment with a physical body for one reason and one reason only, for your learning. It does so happen that under universal law, you learn the fastest and quickest when you are aiding others. In fact, as reasoning man, we must have people around us for we couldn't become enlightened on a desert island. You have to give to others because it is through giving to others that you learn more about reasoning. When you give, you have the opportunity to add to your personal storehouse of knowledge. This is why it is so important to give. All the great spiritual teachers throughout history have led a lifetime of service. They offered their teaching in service to humanity. Each recognized they would complete their education in the physical classroom by aiding others. Why are you in high school? You are there for your learning. Why did you attend grade school? You attended for your learning. Why attend college? The answer is for the learning. If you were going to try to teach the teachers or professors what would be the purpose of attending? Rather, you attend these institutions to further your learning and to learn from those who have gained in understanding of the subject matter. The earth is a schoolroom. When you complete your education in the earthly school, you progress to the next cycle of giving and learning.

When there is no entity in the body, it dies. It is not machines attached to the body which keep it alive and functioning. Left alone by itself without food and attention, the body will cease to function.

Coma is a type of prison. You can't go back and you can't learn anything where you are. It is like being put into solitary confinement. You can't go forward to do what you want with your life. The soul is trapped. You can't use the present to move and learn, nor can you move onto the next step which would be preparing for the next incarnation.

It would be a very unpleasant place to be because the learning opportunities would be very scarce.

By pushing away opportunities for growth, restriction is created. Over time your opportunities become fewer and fewer as you restrict yourself. This is the way a prison is. When you miss out on the ways to be productive in life, you tend to destroy and take, destroy and take. After a while, your world of opportunities gets smaller and smaller until you are in solitary confinement, losing all opportunities in life and eventually dying. You create a specific restriction so that you can learn you have the ability to overcome the limitations of your environment. This usually relates to having passed up opportunities in the past and having restricted your Self. Therefore, there is a need to place your Self in a situation to show or prove to your Self that you have accepted this limitation before.

Any child that rises out of poverty to have great success says, "I will prove to my Self and others I am somebody. I will become more than what my environment says I can become." Have you ever had anybody say to you, "You'll never amount to a hill of beans," or "You can't do that." Later you went on to accomplish that great task, becoming somebody or doing something important. You proved to your Self that you could be more than your environment provided. You can be more than your parents were. That doesn't mean your parents were bad. It means that you can advance beyond your parents' level of learning. You can go beyond their accepted limitations. Regardless of being born into the richest or the poorest family situation, with the kindest or the meanest people, there is an opportunity as long as you are a reasoner, to go beyond the limitations of the environment.

I have been asked, are all pains and aches reversible? I don't know of anyone who has ever had their hand cut off who grew another one. I have heard of sewing hands back on, reattaching them or putting a tooth back in that had been knocked out. But I don't know of anyone who has grown a whole new arm or hand. I believe it is possible. In fact, there are animals that do it. Certain amphibious animals can regrow body appendages. Mankind has not learned to do this yet. For man, regrowth of organs or appendages has not become a part of our evolutionary pattern. There are certain limitations we accept merely by the fact that we are housed in a physical body. As we evolve, the body will also evolve but more importantly we will learn the body is not a limitation.

When people ask, "Is it possible to grow a new leg?" I say, yes, it is possible. Do I think there is anybody in the vicinity who can do it right now? No, I don't. There have probably been individuals throughout history who could accomplish something of this nature, and it is a distinct possibility as man evolves.

Consider the difference between repairing a car engine versus going to a garage and telling a person, "Here is some steel, here is some iron and some metal, plastic, wood, and rubber. Now build an engine." Try telling this to someone who has never built an engine before. It would be impossible for all intents and purposes.

When we have some disorders, to whatever degree, in an organ or part of our body, we want to repair it rapidly in order to stop deterioration and cause quick improvement. It is desirable to cause the body to be in proper balance and full functioning capacity in order that it may serve us. In this manner, the body provides a productive vehicle for man, the inner Self, to learn and develop as a soul.

Often there is the question of young children dying. Parents and friends want to know if a child dies before the age of three, do they have time to learn anything. The answer is yes. There is an inner thinker in a baby's body. The soul brings life force to the body without which it could not exist. The inner thinker also gives attention to the body which it also needs. You know if you walked off and left a car running it would not be long before the engine would cease running for lack of gasoline. Also, if you leave a car out in the open and never start it, it begins to deteriorate. As long as the body is in the mother, it is attached to the umbilical cord and it is living off the energies and fuel of the mother. But once the cord is severed and the baby takes the first breath, then it is leading its own separate existence although it is a dependent existence.

At that point there needs to be attention from the inner Self to the body. When the baby begins to focus the eyesight is when the inner Self resides in the body and has made the full commitment to use the body. There is a real person behind the eyes. This occurs very early in the life of the child and is usually within hours or days of the birth of the child. In the example given of the child with the malformed body, the child can fulfill part of its learning even if the lifetime is a short one such as three years or less. There may be one area of learning that needs fine tuning. Learning needs to be balanced with the older learning. Learning of the quality of love can be practiced enough to add to the whole self in this short time period.

There has to be attention from the inner Self in order for the physical body to be functional. The body has to have a driver. It is as simple as that. Since the soul is providing the driver, which is the inner Self, the conscious mind must give something in return. What is given in return? Permanent learning that we call understanding, stored permanently in the inner Self for all time, is what is given in return. So it is your duty to learn and grow, experience and gain awareness and Self-knowing so you add to the inner Self. Therefore, the duty of the conscious mind is to build wisdom and understanding called permanent learning. A Metaphysical teacher will use all the resources at their command to aid the student in learning permanent healing.

What is a method a teacher of mind and Self could use to aid another to discriminate between the inner and outer mind, particularly if they have a mental handicap? You can start by giving them a puppy to play with. A puppy is something physical that will draw the consciousness or five-sense attention of the child or adult. They will enjoy giving attention to the puppy and it will draw their attention more and more out into the physical environment which is what the introverted individual needs. The puppy provides something physical that can be experienced with the five senses. It has motion that aids the person in giving full attention to the puppy. It would be easier to remove the attention, allowing it to wander, from an inanimate object. You see the puppy. You smell the puppy. You feel the puppy, and you hear the puppy. The puppy is non-threatening, lovable and enjoyable. The puppy provides a reason or purpose for the person to be alive. They have a place to give and receive love.

When you can love the experiences of your life with every ounce of energy you have available right now (mental, emotional, or physical) you are ready for the next stage. Knowing occurs when you practice and apply a new, more expanded way of thinking in your life. Even if a thousand laboratories and a thousand test tubes have proven a theory to be true, <u>you</u> will never know it unless you have directly experienced it with the five senses or with the mind. The words may make sense, you may reason with it and it is all the truth in the world, but as far as making it a permanent part of the inner Self there is always some type of physical practice that needs to occur.

You can read all the best books in the world on riding a bicycle, but when you get on one, you are probably going to fall off a few times. It takes some practice time to master. Collect much information from many difference sources and people who know and have experience in the area about which you desire knowledge. Focus your mind while you are accomplishing the activity so you can begin to perceive mentally what is going on while you are practicing. Instead of depending on the five senses, use the five senses, to learn to perceive with the mind. You can learn to see with your fingers or hear with your eyes. There is a world of difference in the feel of different people who touch you.

The manner in which you embrace your life and the people in your environment, the way you reach out and touch someone instead of seeing the world as something to be feared or something that restricts you, relates to the health of your lungs and respiratory system. The reason the lungs keep filling with mucus when cystic fibrosis is present is due to respiratory diseases and this is connected to the *attitude of restriction, caused by indecision and putting off decisions. A refusal to cause physical action on desires of Self* will cause respiratory difficulties. When the Self refuses to face and use the physical environment, the attention holds onto the past. There may be a desire to live in the present, but there is little effort to cause this to occur.

When a child experiences epileptic seizures there is an emotional overload occurring. For example, a child under seven years of age who has absorbed emotions from the people in his environment and who mentally receives and absorbs thoughts of those around him, can experience an emotional energy overload. This can cause the child to experience a seizure. A child can outgrow this difficulty by learning to form his own thoughts. If the inner thinker is strong, the child learns to develop individual thoughts and attitudes.

At age seven, the child begins to have enough information in the brain so the reasoning process can occur. By this time, the child has learned the attitudes of the parents so that illnesses in many cases are a reflection of the parents' attitudes that the child is absorbing and mimicking. As the child grows older, there is more time to practice limited thinking or to break away from this limited thinking if the child is strong enough and willful enough to do this. At this point the child is making many of his own decisions and formulating those thought patterns himself instead of absorbing them from his environment.

At times a child may develop allergies after a younger sibling is born. How are these two factors connected? When the parents give the younger child much attention, then the older sibling feels that he doesn't have any control in his life and environment. When a younger child has an allergy to food, such as milk, then look to the attitudes of the parents. Look for attitudes, not toward milk, but rather in the way the child limits him Self by allowing the environment to control him. Watch for the way he holds back on saying what is on his mind or expressing what angers him. Identify what he has always wanted to say but never has due to fear. Perceive specifically what he is angry about or afraid of, and what he is holding inside that nobody knows except the child. Remember, the child absorbs the attitudes of the parents.

How to Use This Book

In order to understand an illness or disorder, you will need to find out everything you can about it. Therefore, when an illness or disease presents itself to you or your friends and loved ones, first reference the attitudinal illness section provided in this book, going directly to the section concerned with your specific disorder. Upon reading the attitude-cause and the remedy, you may desire further information. Next, consult the disorder-attitude for illnesses in this area of the body. For example, say you have a cold. First, you read the attitudes and remedy under this section. Next, you remember that when you have had colds in the past it has affected your sinuses, so you turn to *sinus disorders* and read the pertinent information. You also remember at times a cold can be associated with a sore throat. Turn to *throat* in the glossary and read the appropriate attitude and suggestion for remedy.

In addition, recognize a cold affects the respiratory system. Therefore, you may want to look up *respiratory system* and read the cause, which is a mental attitude disorder, as well as the remedy or suggestions for improvement.

Remember, the sinus area, throat, and respiratory attitudes will hold secondary importance to those given under the first category known as *cold*. This is because this encyclopedia of disease-attitude remedies is <u>specific</u>. If you have a specific pain, illness, or disorder there exists a <u>specific</u> attitude, a habitual thought pattern, producing the disorder.

The important point to remember is that the human body is not a group of isolated parts. Rather, the body is designed to function as a whole unit with every part working together and in harmony for the total well-being of the whole. Therefore, whenever an organ, gland, or area of the body is experiencing pain, discomfort, or ill health, that section of the body will also affect other areas. In fact, it will affect the system as a whole. The common cold may affect the sinuses but it also affects the whole body, leaving you feeling achy all over.

Stress is a term that has come into common usage recently to indicate that the mind of the individual does in fact have a causal effect on the bodily health. However, we can and must go far beyond this generalized and simple truth. We must realize that for every illness in the body there is a causal mental action and that cause is you. You create and affect your body every single day, mentally, emotionally, and physically.

Do not underestimate this. Every thought you have has reality. Thoughts have energy and are real. Thoughts repeated for a length of time gain in power and force, gradually making themselves more and more known in our everyday life.

When an unproductive thought pattern is produced continuously for weeks, months, or sometimes even years, it can have far reaching effects. The physical body can begin to show the effect physically of the emotional and mental wear and tear. Soon, the weak link in the body snaps or breaks down and we have what is known as dis-ease or illness in the body.

The physical body has many systems. Some of these are the endocrine system, the nervous system, the skeletal system, the muscular system, the reproductive system, the cardiovascular system, the lymphatic system, the respiratory system, the urinary system, and the digestive system. A specific mental attitude is necessary to create disorder in each of these areas.

For example, the specific attitude that creates disorders in the digestive system is a refusal to embrace situations occurring in the life. This attitude creates a limitation in one's ability to gain knowledge and Self awareness. If we want to further identify a specific area of the digestive system such as the intestines as the center of the physical disorder, we move through the glossary of disorders locating the word *intestines*. To the right of the physical disorder is the associated attitude which is, *"holding on to or rejecting ideas whether past or present opinions"*.

It is easy to see how a refusal to use the present, due to mentally living in the past and replaying in the mind painful experiences from an earlier point in your life, will align with the attitude which creates disorders in the digestive system, *"a refusal to utilize situations in the present for learning and assimilation of experiences."*

Another part of the digestive system is the gall bladder. The attitude associated with gall bladder difficulties is *"trying to control others due to a fear of being controlled and a fear of being out of control."* If one is to live in fear, then the fear is what one will create. The fear of being out of control and/or trying to control others translates into difficulty in using each experience every day as an opportunity for Self improvement and Self fulfillment. Put another way, if you are afraid of people, then all of your attention is on this fear leaving little or no time for learning, sharing and Self fulfillment.

The stomach provides another example of how one area of the body system with an attitude disorder can relate to the whole system. The unproductive attitude associated with stomach disorders is *difficulty in receiving new information.* This in turn is due to thinking of unplesant events that could possibly happen in the future. We call this type of thinking, worry. When one's attention is on creating mental pictures of what you do <u>not</u> want to occur in the future, then there is very little or ineffective use of the present situation. Therefore there is little learning and growth in the present.

Consider the case of the attitude associated with the liver which plays a vital role in the digestive process. The unproductive thought pattern associated with the liver is *an attitude of worthlessness* and *a need to create a purpose in life.* Again associating this attitude with the whole, it is very difficult to learn, grow and utilize any experience where there is an absence of self worth. Self value is the foundation on which we build our whole lives.

The attitude associated with that part of the digestive system known as the pancreas also connects with the attitude for the digestive system. When disorders occur in the pancreas, they are due to *restricted giving.* In order to learn and gain from our experiences in life, it is necessary to give to others and remove the selfishness. As we give to others we create a space within ourselves so we may receive. Until we are ready to receive and have deemed ourselves worthy of receiving, there is no way we can create, learn, and grow. The process of maturing as a creator is one of giving to others in the environment in order that we may receive in return. The greatest gift we can give is our Selves. Clear, honest, open, and deep communication is one of the highest forms of giving one can attain. It provides the opportunity for some of the greatest learning.

The endocrine system provides another example of how you may use this book both with the specific area of the body in which you experience discomfort and also to note associated and generalized unproductive attitudes working with the entire system.

Now suppose if you are female you have a disorder in the ovaries or, if you are male, a difficulty concerning the testicles. You look up the disorder in the glossary provided in this book finding the mental attitude for the ovaries relates to *difficulty in use and power of the feminine expression and receptivity*, while for the male the attitude is a *difficulty with the masculine expression and a misunderstanding of aggressiveness.*

Suppose you desire to understand more about creating and the essence of sexuality. In your research you discover the ovaries and testicles are part of the endocrine system. The thought pattern concerned with the endocrine system is *difficulties with change in regards to the transformation of energies*. This thought attitude is linked with the creative ability and the need to move forward with one's creations both aggressively and receptively. The two factors of any creation are the aggressive quality which means to initiate and sustain activity, and the receptive quality which is to open one Self to receive with the whole mind and being.

Also included in the endocrine system are the pituitary and thyroid glands. The thyroid, adrenals and gonads are mediated and influenced by the hormones of the pituitary gland. Hormones affect the activity of tissues within the body. These hormones can enter the bloodstream affecting the entire body. Hormones adjust the equilibrium in the body enabling it to respond to the stresses of life in a coordinated manner. Many times when one of these is affected, it will in turn affect the ovaries and testicles as these are part of the same system. The pituitary gland's associated attitude is *the need to use the thinking process productively*. To focus one's attention and to visualize goals and ideals for one's life is a must in order to reason and be the cause of one's life. Without the thinking process being used effectively, little or no creation can occur which is the overall theme of the endocrine system.

In a similar connected fashion, the mental attitude disorder of the thyroid influences the capabilities of the endocrine system. *Will* is the connecting attitude associated with the thyroid gland. A misuse of will affects the thyroid gland, for you see without will, the ability to choose and act, there can be no creation. The attitude-disorder affecting the endocrine system is an *impairment in creating or creation.* Reasoning and will are required for the thinker to create and build, to add to and improve.

Today, heart attacks and vascular problems are major diseases for thousands of people. The cardiovascular system provides the important duty of supplying the body with life-giving blood and carrying away toxins and impurities from the system. This system includes the heart as well as the veins and arteries. Arteries leave the heart and connect to the organs of the body. Veins leave the organs to return blood to the heart.

Today, many people are worried about the condition of their heart. When difficulties with the heart are present, there is an attitude that *responsibility is a burden.* There is a misunderstanding of responsibility as a burden. Often there is the mistaken belief that it is one's responsibility to keep up with friends, family, and neighbors in the amount of possessions one can accumulate. This competition with others for specific material possessions is often in direct conflict with what one actually wants to achieve in life. This discontent in leading a double life results in conflicting signals to the body that may eventually result in heart disorders, including heart attacks.

Difficulty with the veins of the body, for example varicose veins, is the result of an attitude of *difficulty with responsibility or responding to conditions* to the point that little forward motion is produced in the life.

The life energy is distributed by the blood to the various parts of the body. The heart acts as the pump for the circulation of this energy. The blood system responds to the needs of the body.

Nervous system disorders affect many people no matter what their age or background. The nervous system consists of the brain, spinal cord, and peripheral nerves. Difficulties occurring in the nervous system indicate *a need to give attention to receiving and using information productively* which requires directed attention. When a person refuses to create a purpose for living, there is little correct use of the senses in gathering input, therefore, the nerves and nerve endings begin to deteriorate. The solution to correct this condition is to set new goals with new purposes in life. Seek out new exciting and fun adventures. Initiate action on that desire you have been putting off for so long. Listen to your inner urge, your inner bliss that nudges you to try something new.

The brain is also considered part of the nervous system. Images, impressions, and inputs received through the nerves and sensory organs are transferred to the brain. The brain processes the information it receives, correlating it with previously stored information called memory. Then plans are created for future strategies of action. This is called imagination.

Difficulties in the brain arise from *misuse or incomplete use of the thinking process*. Scattered attention or incomplete use of imagination has major effects on this area. The brain is dependent on the nerves to supply it with information and experience in order for reasoning to occur. Therefore, recognize that controlled and directed use of the attention is of primary importance in improving and maintaining any area of the nervous system.

The skeletal system consists of the many bones of the physical body, including the cranium, the spinal column and vertebrae, and the pelvis. The skeletal system provides the structural framework for the body. Difficulties and disorders in the skeletal system will relate to an attitude of thinking *Self is incapable of using structure to cause forward motion in the life.* This structure may be your job, club, organization, or marriage for each of these require a structure in order to function.

The lymphatic system provides a defense system for the body against virus, bacteria, aches, and pains. *An attitude of defensiveness or thinking one is incapable of fulfilling desires* will feed a signal to the lymphatic system that it constantly needs to be at work defending the body. The overworking of the lymphatic system causes a wearing out and weakening in the area. This weakening gives an avenue of entry for microorganisms. Then one gets frequent colds, sinusitis, influenza, or other microbial dis-eases.

Comprehensive Survey of Mind-Body Relationship

You will notice in reading through the glossary of physical disorders and related mental attitude causes that from time to time an attitude will be associated with two or more physical illnesses. The first reaction may be to think, how can this be if this book is specific? The answer is that in most cases the illnesses are related. For example, the mental attitude producing inflammation is *anger and an over-reaction to outer or inner environment due to defensiveness.* Notice also that abscess has listed *suppressed anger* as the mental attitude disorder. On closer examination, we find an abscess to be a localized collection of pus, the result of disintegration of tissue. Inflammation is often encountered when we have an abscess.

You may after consideration of the matter come to the conclusion as I have, that anger is a localized collection of unproductive thoughts and emotions which is the result of the disintegration of what previously was a more productive structure of mind, thought, and attitude.

Another example of related mental attitudes creating relative physical disorders can be traced to skin disorders, particularly acne. Read the mental attitude for the disorder of acne. This is *dislike for one's own expression.* Now read the attitude for the face: *hiding one's identity and creating a fake identity.* Consider that dislike for the way one expresses Self to others shows either one does not like who he is (identity) and so, like an adolescent, he must pretend to be something he is not in order to have the approval of peers or he may feel incapable due to lack of experience of expressing his real Self.

The skin serves as the outer covering of our body and as such it represents the manner in which we present our inner Selves to the world. When skin disorders are present, they are an indication one is not at peace with the manner in which he presents himself outwardly to the world.

Melanoma is a malignancy of the skin and is created by *a distaste or disgust for the image one has of the Self.* Its attitudinal cause is similar to the overall attitude causing cancer of the skin which is *hatred for the way one presents Self outwardly to others.*

Scleroderma falls under the same category of attitudes affecting the skin. In this case, the attitude is *defensiveness that is practiced in the way one expresses to another.* Many times this person will be gruff and overbearing, directing their anger outwardly at others.

The mental attitude for the disorder of an excessive appetite is *having desires you want to fulfill but feeling you can't have those desires.* Compare this with the thought processes involved with being overweight which is due to *unfulfilled desires.* Therefore, you see that an attitude which produces an excessive appetite leads to an overweight body thus perpetuating a vicious cycle that is often difficult to break.

Asthma is an illness of major proportion. Many people who have asthma feel they have to live with it for the rest of their lives. Asthma is created by *denying the desires of Self.* There is a fear of loss of freedom that comes from feeling trapped and that one is incapable of fulfilling one's own desires.

Compare the mental attitude disorder for asthma with that of bronchitis. The common thread is once again the true desires of Self are not being fulfilled. However, with bronchitis there is the additional factor of *blaming others for one's own lack of desire fulfillment.* It is the blame and the resulting anger which create the inflammation associated with bronchitis.

The mental attitude disorder resulting in respiratory system problems is *restriction creating emotional repression from not fulfilling desires.* There is usually a lack of verbalizing the real, true, and often secret desires of one Self. This creates restriction. Our physical bodies need air to sustain life. Without air or oxygen we would not survive very long, therefore, mental restriction often shows up in the respiratory system first.

The common cold will often restrict the breath and clog the respiratory system. The thought pattern called *indecision* restricts for if one refuses to choose, there can be no movement forward towards one's goals thus stifling the ability to receive. This creates restriction.

Mononucleosis is also the result of indecision, but with the specificity of having been practiced over a long period of time over a particular issue.

At times when the lymphatic system is weak or in disarray, the attitude of *defensiveness and self pity* is present. The thought of being *powerless to cause change* is present as well. This attitude weakens the immune system. Such a person may see himself as a child who is at the mercy of the adults in the environment for his wants, needs, and protection. Sinusitis fits into this category. The attitude-cause for sinusitis is *self pity* that results from a refusal to cause any productive change in the life. Therefore you feel sorry for yourself. Following the self pity in many cases is anger. This is similar to a child throwing a temper tantrum, the "poor me" syndrome.

An individual is made more susceptible to infections when he is being defensive. Why would one be defensive? Because the time, effort, and attention needed to cause forward motion and the fulfillment of desires is absent. This attitude of defensiveness wears down and weakens the immune system, reducing its efficiency in resisting disease.

For example, influenza and the common cold are created by indecisiveness. When an individual is indecisive, he or she is sitting on the fence which produces no motion, no learning, no-thing. When the body is not exercised it becomes weak. When the mind is not exercised through willful decision-making it also becomes weak. Have you ever noticed that you feel the need to defend yourself the most when you are feeling weak and in a precarious, insecure position? When you are strong, confident, and secure, you do not defend, rather you command, and express the value of what you are doing. You aggressively move forward in life and in the fulfillment of your creations. Indecisiveness leaves a person weak, making them easy prey for a host of microorganisms that lead to colds, influenza, and other viral and bacterial infections. With this information in hand you can begin to strengthen yourself and lead a healthier and more invigorating life.

Consider the dis-ease known as cancer and the many areas of the body in which it may arise. The reader will observe cancer to be caused by *hatred of Self*. Sometimes this hatred is expressed only inwardly, or you may know people who express anger and rage toward others in their environment. After determining the area of the body in which the cancer is located, one may specify and isolate the source of the hatred. Cancer of the uterus will show a female who hates being female, or hates how she thinks she has been abused as a female, or hates using the receptive quality. The same will hold true for a male who has prostate cancer except the hate will revolve around his masculinity and hatred of the aggressive quality. Both will show a need to use the creative potential within oneself.

Cancer of the liver will demonstrate a hatred for life or a hatred that one has not fulfilled their purpose or assignment in life. Cancer of the lungs is caused from a hatred of the way one has restricted himself and postponed desires in life. Cancer of the gall bladder is created when one hates not having the control in life and not being able to control others. Cancer of the stomach is produced when one hates living in the present situations and circumstances while doing little to change them. Cancer of the pancreas comes from hatred of giving. Cancer of the throat is developed when an individual hates to exercise their will to change or move forward in life.

Tumors, when malignant, are caused by *hatred*. When benign, they are created by *unproductive concentrated thoughts* other than hatred. Hatred is one of the most damaging of all unproductive attitudes because it can completely direct one away from his true assignment in life.

In following the theme of this chapter, connecting related unproductive thought attitudes to related areas of the body, consider the intestinal system and its various parts. Difficulties in the intestinal area are related to *an attitude of holding onto the past*. This translates into a refusal to use the present effectively for much of one's attention remains in the past. At times, a person with this problem may seem to reject his own past whereas in reality he is avoiding looking at some pain associated with the past and is therefore a slave to it.

The mental attitude disorder for colon problems is *holding on to the past* which is consistent with disorders in the intestines. Holding onto the past interferes with using the present effectively in much the same way as feeling guilty or being angry about something about the past while eating can give one indigestion and interfere with the proper assimilation of foods. Indigestion can be created by giving one's attention to something other than the food being eaten. This attention may be on memory of the past or in the imagination.

Disorders in the pituitary may be compared and contrasted with difficulties in the ovaries or testicles for all are part of the endocrine system and thus are connected by an attitude of difficulty with change in regards to the transformation of energies. The ovaries and testicles reflect the *misuse of receptivity and the aggressive quality respectively*. All of these are indispensable for creation. The thyroid's associative attitude of use or misuse of will provides a required factor of creation. For any creation to occur one must make a decision and act on it. In fact, impotence is manifested from *insecurity in responding when the aggressive quality is required*.

Eye problems show an indication of *difficulty with using mental perception*. Recognize each eye disorder will fall under this general category. Farsightedness will relate to *clouding of one's perception from refusing to use the present due to rejecting new ideas and input received each day*. Nearsightedness is brought about when the individual has a *vagueness in creating goals*. This usually occurs when all the individual's attention is on the present and what is right in front of him with little regard for tomorrow. It can indicate a rejection of the future. An example of this is when a person sees the future as being gloomy.

Anemia is brought about through *thinking of Self as incapable of fulfilling one's desires* which is closely related to blood disorders in general created by an attitude of Self weakness in responding to life. A generalized, unproductive attitude becomes specific to an individual and this in turn creates specific types of blood disorders. Also compare with the attitude causing disorders in the arteries which is *the need to respond to stimulus and thinking responsibility is a burden*.

Difficulties with the heart and heart disease are disorders of strong interest to many people. The heart is an integral part of the circulatory system. It is the pump for the blood circulating through the body. Heart disorders are often created through a *misunderstanding of responsibility*. Perhaps, a person may feel it is his responsibility to have a car that is as luxurious and expensive as his neighbors. He may think he must have a large house with a two-car garage, the latest television, video and audio equipment as well as a boat or yacht. He purchases these items, not because he desires or even needs them. Rather, this type of individual buys them to maintain the status quo, "to keep up with the Joneses", and to maintain his public image.

However, the real competition is not with others for trying to possess objects just because others say that is what you should do is practicing misplaced responsibility. Responsibility is always first and foremost to one's learning and growth. When one is gaining new awarenesses and discoveries about Self, life is exciting and a person experiences a sense of fulfillment. When one's attention is solely on pleasing others, then life loses its meaning. Others' desires may be different from your own. To live your life as an adult based on others' desires is somewhat ludicrous for it leads to a sad, unfulfilling life.

The sadness created from leading a false life, one that is different or opposed to your own desires, creates a weakening of the body as the life force or inner strength of the thinker is weakened by the unwillingness to respond to one's own desires. This weakening caused by a misunderstanding of the ability to respond to one's own desires called "response-ability" is reflected in difficulties in the heart and circulatory system. This system distributes the life-carrying blood throughout the body bringing with it oxygen and nutrition. It also carries off waste and toxins from the system, ensuring the body is maintained. When a person refuses to give attention to his inner desires, the result is unhappiness and a sense that something is missing in life. When the attention is only directed towards pleasing others and their desires, the heart and circulatory system may be harmed.

For those of you who, after reading these words, say to your Selves, "Well, isn't that very selfish to think of your Self first?" I say you must take care of your health and happiness first if you are going to help others. In truth, the better person you become, the better position from which you can help others. A healthy, intelligent person who loves Self and who has developed some wealth is in the best position to give of love and possessions as well as high quality time and attention to others. In order to heal others, we must heal our Selves. In order to love others, we must learn to love our Selves. In order to give consistently to others, we must give to our Selves.

Stroke is related to the blood and circulatory system. It affects the brain. Due to these factors, the mental attitude cause may be traced to a combination of factors. Stroke is created by a *refusal to face or respond to conditions and experiences within one's life.* Avoidance of conditions, circumstances, or learning in the life is irresponsible. The responsibility factor or the need to respond is the connecting link between stroke and heart attack. Stroke is created by a refusal to respond, whereas, heart attack is created as a person misdirects his own responsiveness to living his life according to other people's desires and ideas of how he should live his life.

Stroke, being associated with the head area carries the additional factors of the need to use all aspects of reasoning. Some of these qualities are imagination and perception. The person who creates stroke has stopped living his dreams. He has created excuses for not fulfilling his dreams and for staying exactly the way he is, keeping his life as it is with no movement toward his goals and ideals.

Lack of motion producing little growth in the life due to one's Self-imposed limitations causes many millions to suffer from difficulties with joints in the body, particularly arthritis. Disorders restricting the motion of the joints are a result of *mental restriction.* Imagine living in a self-imposed prison of your own attitudes. Four walls and narrowly confined space leave little room for the freedom of learning and growth. In a prison someone else determines when and what you will eat. They decide what you will wear, what you will read, and who you will talk to. In short, your freedom is severely restricted. Limited, negative or unproductive thinking results in missed opportunities and a reduced freedom of response to life's wonders. In other words, restriction.

Arthritis is the effect of the *mental restrictions placed on one's Self.* If you have difficulties in the joints then practice listening to all the times you say the words, "I can't" or "I cannot." A not is no-thing. "Should not, could not, would not, can not, will not, may not," are all ways of negating one's own life as well as the opportunities life presents. Saying

NO when an opportunity arises for learning a new skill or ability, or saying NO to an opportunity to give to another only restricts and retards one's own life and pushes farther into the future the day when one will be enlightened. Arthritis proceeds from an "I can't" or "I am not able or not capable" attitude in the present.

When the limitations of the Self are created from *condemning one's Self for past mistakes and errors*, the effect is to harm the kidneys and urinary system. Problems in the kidneys are related to difficulties in the urinary system of which they are a part. The attitude that causes dysfunction in the urinary system is *regret and guilt*. Regret is grief or pain associated with the past. Disappointment and remorse are also a part of regret.

When kidney problems arise, guilt and condemnation are the culprits. Both of these attitudes relate to a need to stop beating yourself up due to a mistake or mistakes made in the past. Instead of blaming your Self, look for the cause. Learn from the experience in order that you will not repeat the same mistake. If you learn from a mistake, then it was not a failure. It was a learning experience!

This chapter was designed with the intention of aiding the reader in his or her use of the attitudes-physical disorder glossary. My goal in sharing this research is to educate the world by presenting the interconnectedness of the whole being, mentally, emotionally, and physically, not only for the physical body and its systems but also for the unproductive mental attitudes that cause these disorders.

Imagine the tremendous advantage you have by using this information. If a symptom shows itself in your body, you immediately have access to the thought pattern producing the difficulty. You can cross reference and gain additional insight. You may use the suggestions for improvement if you are at a loss as to where to begin. Imagine a world where the question, "Why did this happen to me?" could be answered by each of its inhabitants when they develop an illness.

This education is of paramount importance in our evolutionary drive for understanding our Selves, the environment in which we live, and to bring about world peace. World peace will only occur as peace is developed in the individuals who make up humanity.

Every time an ache or pain, disease, disorder, or illness in your body presents itself you may use this book as an aid in identifying your own unproductive thoughts and attitudes. The more people are aware of their own shortcomings and change them, adapt and grow, the greater will the total resources of our community, country and planet be. There is such a relief in knowing the cause of a physical effect in your life for only then do you begin to really and truly have control.

Some of you will have a disorder, will read the mental attitude cause of this disorder and say to your Self and others, "this is not me, this cannot possibly be me, I don't think like that." To these people I present several suggestions. The *first* is to go to friends and acquaintances, people you can count on to be honest and straightforward with you even to the point of hurting your feelings. Relate to these people the mental attitude disorder presented in this book for your physical illness. Then ask these people, "Am I really like that, and do I do these things mentioned?" The answer will be very illuminating.

Second, I suggest you write the mental attitude disorder on paper and carry that paper with you every day for one month. Read this paper first thing upon arising in the morning, at lunch time, and immediately before retiring to bed at night. This process will place the knowledge so firmly in your mind that when your thoughts or your actions match the attitude-disorder listed, you will recognize it immediately. You will experience the freedom of gaining greater Self realization and you are to be congratulated for your efforts. You are now in a much better position to aid others also.

A *third* suggestion, is to read the mental attitude, and meditate on it for at least 15 minutes a day for a month.

A *fourth* suggestion, is to use suggestions for improvement given in the glossary every day for a month. Log in the journal how you have used the suggestion listed. At the end of one month, review the log and summarize. In this manner, you will come to realize the ways you have limited your Self in the past. You will then experience the excitement of knowing you can now do more with your life and be more than you had ever before thought possible.

Visualization and Affirmation

Visualization is a powerful tool that you will be using in creating a happier, healthier, and more prosperous you.

The essence of visualization is thought. In fact, visualization is controlled, directed thought. What is thought? Thought is a mental picture, created and held within a mind. Thought is a mental picture. Read the word *elephant*. You will notice that you created a mental picture in your mind's eye of what an elephant looks and acts like. This is true for the word *car, airplane, house,* or *clothes*. Each of these words creates a different picture on our mental movie screen.

Words, and in fact, all languages, are methods of describing mental pictures so we may share our thoughts with others.

Over the years of our lives, we had created certain compulsive ways of thinking. These ways or manners of thinking create repetitive thought pictures in mind. These repetitive thought pictures when unproductive or limiting create trouble in our waking life which we term pain.

In life, we are either creating and producing or using up and tearing down, for, you see, the nature of the physical is change. We must learn to use change productively, in order to have a satisfying and meaningful life.

Create a mental picture in your mind's eye with the words *love, compassion, caring, courage, strength, integrity, dignity, value,* and *respect*. These words create a mental idea or thought of wholeness, harmony, productivity, aiding others, and a valuable existence.

Now create a mental picture in your mind's eye with the words *hate, resentment, guilt, worry, fear, disrespect, condemnation,* and *anger.* Notice what a different mental picture these words stimulate in relation to the first group of words. The second group of words such as *hate, resentment* and *anger,* create mental pictures of destruction and tearing down what has already been produced.

This is exactly what unproductive attitudes produce in our bodies and life; destructiveness and tearing down of what has already been produced.

An attitude is a thought pattern repeatedly and consistently created in the mind by the individual. The mind is a vehicle for the individual, the thinker, to use. It needs to be used wisely. Unproductive attitudes of hate, guilt, or fear tear down the same body that the individual has spent years producing. Therefore, we must replace unproductive thoughts and attitudes with thoughts that have creative strength.

Visualization provides a method, an avenue, of learning to consciously and willfully create productive thought pictures to replace unproductive or limiting concepts.

Visualization has its limitations though. It does little good to visualize a healthy body for five or ten minutes a day and then spend the rest of the day being resentful towards someone because they are not behaving as you would desire them to whether it is your wife, husband, brother, employer, friend, enemy, or child.

We must learn to create and maintain the positive, productive mental pictures throughout the day, week, and year if we are to create and maintain a healthy, productive, and useful body. This was the lesson I learned as a child over thirty years ago. It has served me well.

A good first step is to practice concentration. First, you gain the ability to hold your attention on productive thoughts and experiences in order to derive the most benefit from them, and secondly through the practice of concentration the individual gains awareness of his thoughts. This is the first step of Self awareness. Through awareness of our thoughts, we gain the freedom of choosing the thoughts and mental pictures we desire to maintain.

All creation begins with thought. Creating the more productive rest of your life entails beginning now to create more positive and productive thought pictures.

An affirmation provides a short-term stimulus for a certain desired thought picture. It provides value if the person will take the time and attention to create a mental picture of what the words represent. This productive mental picture must then be practiced over and over in order to have permanent lasting effects.

I personally practiced visualization for over an hour a day for many years. I experienced tremendous benefits. However, the greatest benefit was in learning to hold the mental pictures I desired at all times.

PERMANENT HEALING
Section II

GLOSSARY

Physical Disorders
Mental Attitude Disorders
Suggestions for Improvement

Problem *Physical Disorder*	**Cause** *Mental Attitude Disorder*
Abdominal Pain	Desire for attention from others.
Abrasion	Scattered attention.
Abscess	Suppressed anger.
Accidents	Neglect in how one uses the attention.
Aches (pains)	Depends on area producing pain. See specific area.
Achilles Tendon	Straining or forcing the body rather than using mental direction. Thinking of the Self as physical.
Acne	Dislike for one's own expression.
Addictions	Fear of being able to stand on one's own. Idea of powerlessness. Dependency.
drugs	Wanting to escape from facing Self.
Addison's Disease *see: Adrenal Problems*	Suppression of emotions, particularly anger.

Remedy *Suggestions for Improvement*	*Personal Notes* *& Observations*
Use the experience for learning.	
Learn to control and focus the attention.	
Each day look at your Self in a mirror and state out loud your thoughts and feelings.	
Concentrate on an object of your choice for ten minutes each day. For example, use the tip of your finger, the end of a pen or pencil or a dot on the wall.	
Create a clear picture of your next goal. Initiate immediate and regular, day-by-day, step-by-step action on this goal.	
Study and develop mental power.	
Communicate and express yourSelf until you like and enjoy the expression of Self. Share the Self in communication and you will appreciate Self value.	
Begin to accept responsibility for your life by admitting you have caused your Self to be this way. Now love your Self enough to change.	
Practice meditation daily in order to meet and come to know your true, valuable Self. Learn to interpret your dreams in order that you may understand the subconscious mind naturally.	
Share your feelings with others. Open up and be honest with what you are experiencing inside so your emotions do not become blown out of proportion.	

Problem *Physical Disorder*	**Cause** *Mental Attitude Disorder*
Adenoids	Self pity. Going over information in the thoughts about what can be productive without any intention to change, which is a misuse of the will.
Adrenal Problems *see: Addison's Disease, Cushing's Disease*	Emotional repression, particularly in regard to reacting with fear rather than causing desire.
Aging Problems	Refusal to change from desire. Refusal or difficulty in setting goals. Regret (attention in past on opportunities that have been lost or not used) without attention being given to the present on how learning can occur and how situations in life can be used.
AIDS	Resentment of one's identity and expression. An attitude that others are against you. Rebellion. Misplaced attempt to get even with someone.
Alcoholism *see: Drug Addictions*	Attitude of worthlessness.
Allergies *see: Hay Fever*	Mental oversensitivity to one's environment, particularly people. Thinking Self is vulnerable to others.
Alzheimer's Disease *see: Dementia, Senility*	Difficulty in imagining the future and a desire to return to childhood. Desire to remain in the past and feeling useless in the present.

Remedy *Suggestions for Improvement*	*Personal Notes* *& Observations*
Make five decisions each day and produce action on them by exercising will. Imagine your Self doing the activity you want and being the person you want to be.	
In most situations, there are more than just two choices. You can do more than fight or run away. You can verbalize with emotion your productive desires and insights. Always give of your Self instead of worrying about other's reactions.	
Turn a desire into a goal to accomplish each day. You have a lifetime of valuable learning and experience, and there is no substitute for experience. Share your wisdom with others. Be a resource others can use.	
Make your thoughts and words to match. Cause your thoughts, words, and deeds to be in alignment. Practice Self honesty.	
Set one goal with a benefit for Self each day and make it happen. To establish worthiness in yourself, initiate one action each day on what you believe to be worthy and valuable.	
Say what is on your mind with good intentions. Act on your desires. Create and set aside a time each day for an activity you enjoy such as a hobby, reading, or writing.	
Set daily, weekly, monthly, yearly, and lifetime goals. Fulfill the desire you have postponed for years, such as visiting a country or city, writing a book, or singing in a choir.	

Problem *Physical Disorder*	**Cause** *Mental Attitude Disorder*
Amenorrhea see: *Female Problems, Menstrual Problems*	Fear of maturing, rejection of the feminine expression.
Amnesia	Refusal to face the truth.
Amyotrophic Lateral Sclerosis (Lou Gehrig's Disease)	Attachment to a particular identity that has changed. Attachment to what the individual thinks has been lost.
Anemia see: *Bleeding*	Thinking of Self as incapable of responding to and fulfilling one's desires.
Angina	Fear of not being able to fulfill one's responsibilities.
Ankles	Need to give attention to one's body. Being discouraged due to obligations made that are no longer desired.
Anorectal Bleeding	Forcing or straining with ideas caused by refusing the release the past.
Anorexia	Refusal to grow up, to learn and mature.
Anus see: *Hemorrhoids*	Seeing the past as being the cause or blame for what is seen as failure in the present. Holding onto the past with regret or blame which creates a forcing type of attitude in the present.

Remedy *Suggestions for Improvement*	*Personal Notes* *& Observations*
Grow up. Start loving your Self enough to be an adult. Responsibility means the ability to respond and is the definition of freedom.	
Be honest with your Self and others. Admit the truth outwardly. State: "I created my life the way it is, therefore, I can make it the way I desire."	
You can't be who you were yesterday, so formulate your idea of the new you. You are not a job, you are not a body, you are a soul inhabiting a body.	
You really can have anything you desire. Believe in yourself. Begin work on your fondest desires. The universe is yours to use.	
Make sure some action is taken towards your personal goals each day, no matter how small or how large.	
Appreciate the body as the temple of the real Self. Realize you still can fulfill your desires and create meaning in life. It is not too late.	
Stop procrastinating. Create a clear mental picture of your goal and desire, acting on this each day.	
Grow up. Read about and observe successful people. Discover their valuable qualities and attributes. Make those valuable qualities a part of Self.	
Create a door and doorway to your desires. Now open it. You don't need to break the door down.	

Problem *Physical Disorder*	**Cause** *Mental Attitude Disorder*
abscess	Repression of thoughts particularly those having to do with past mistakes.
bleeding *see: Anorectal Bleeding*	
fistula	same
Anxiety	Scattered attention.
Aorta	Ignoring that the purpose of existence or life is learning.
Apathy	No goals. Therefore there is no purpose either.
Appendicitis	Desire for attention but a fear of sudden change. Repressed ideas of dissatisfaction with the environment. Rebellion against information coming from sources outside of Self. This causes an explosion in the body.
Appetite excessive	Having desires you want to fulfill but feeling you can't have those desires. Accepting second best.
loss *see: Anorexia*	Refusal to nurture your Self, mentally, emotionally, or spiritually.

Remedy *Suggestions for Improvement*	*Personal Notes* *& Observations*
Talk with others about the pains of the past until the pain subsides. Prove to your Self that you are more today than you were yesterday by creating on a grander scale. Improve on what is.	
Give your full attention to everyone you meet and those in your environment. Love and care enough about everything you do and everyone's life you touch to give your whole mind and attention.	
Your greatest responsibility is to your Self and that responsibility is to cause permanent learning, permanent growth in you each day.	
Find some activity not related to your job and make time each day to have fun with that activity.	
Make small changes in your life each day. Wear different clothes, drive a different route to work, take a bus, read a different subject in a magazine. Look for ways to expand your Self.	
You must prove to Self you can fulfill your personal desires by extending your Self with will power beyond previously accepted limitations.	
Do something just for Self each day.	

Problem *Physical Disorder*	**Cause** *Mental Attitude Disorder*
Arm(s)	Lack of purpose or mobility of purpose. Need to initiate the aggressive action of responding to a stimulus.
Arteries	Attitude that responsibility is a burden.
Arteriosclerosis	Prejudice. Feeling responsible for living up to others' expectations. Constantly comparing the Self in a negative sense to others. Rigidity in thinking regarding any type of idea that has been formed. Difficulty in receiving new information.
Arthritis see: *Joints*	Restrictions placed upon Self.
Asphyxiating Attacks see: *Breathing Problems, Hyperventilation*	Fear of not being able to fulfill the desires of the Self.
Asthma	Denial of desires of Self. Fear of loss of freedom. Feeling trapped by thinking Self is repeating mistakes. Thinking Self is incapable of fulfilling the desires.
Athlete's Foot see: *Foot*	
Avarice	Thinking that others can take from Self.

Remedy *Suggestions for Improvement*	*Personal Notes* *& Observations*
Create some type of personal benefit for the things you do each day. Listen to the inner voice, the inner bliss, that is saying, "This is what I really want to do with my life."	
Recognize responsibility and burden are not synonymous. Your ability to respond to your desires is what creates freedom of motion for you.	
Same as above. In addition, realize the reason you are in this life is for your learning and growth. As you learn and grow you are able to help many more people and still not restrict your freedom.	
Push beyond the limitations you have imagined for your Self. Know what you want and don't take no for an answer.	
Initiate one step each day toward one of your desires. The little steps, practiced consistently, create the bigger steps and the fulfillment of your desires.	
You gain control by creating a clear, mental picture of what you want to think, say, or do. Make sure you cause your picture to become a physical reality. Speak and say what is on your mind. Tell everyone you meet exactly what you would like to be doing with your life.	
Learn how to give.	

Problem *Physical Disorder*	**Cause** *Mental Attitude Disorder*
Back *see: Area of Back, Spinal Misalignments*	Difficulty in knowing how to be flexible in responding to change. Creates a feeling of loss of control or powerlessness.
cranial	Feeling pressured by external factors.
lumbar (lower)	Activity. Difficulties exercising one's own power and authority. Thinking others are in control of Self.
thoracic (middle)	Purpose. Fear or apprehension of the ability to cause what is desired in the life.
cervical (upper)	Ideal. Worry. Attention is on what Self does not want to occur. Misplaced responsibility, feeling responsible for others rather than Self.
Bad Breath *see: Halitosis, Digestion*	
Balance, Loss of (Inner Ear)	Refusing to hear or listen to Self or environment.
Baldness	Procrastination in fulfilling desires. Chronic refusal to make decisions or pursue the many ideas and desires of Self.
Bedwetting	Fear of being out of control. Fear of ridicule.

Remedy *Suggestions for Improvement*	*Personal Notes & Observations*
Willingly create changes and improvement in the life each day. Do not settle for living the life habitually.	
Maintain attention on your desires and be determined to achieve them.	
Direct your Self and your energy. Your thoughts and ideas have value. Share them with others and teach the value you have to offer.	
You can accomplish anything you desire when you put your mind to it. Step forward each day.	
You are responsible for your Self. By responding to your desires, you can aid others to a greater degree.	
Practice meditation every day. Remember and write down your dreams every morning upon arising. Both meditation and dreams are tools for listening to your inner Self.	
Stop putting off life and pretending to be something you are not. Instead, communicate your real thoughts and feelings with others and be honest with your expression of desires.	
Choose a condition you want to create each day.	

Problem *Physical Disorder*	**Cause** *Mental Attitude Disorder*
Belching	Attitude of being deprived.
Bigotry	Need to build will power and desires of Self.
Birth Defects *see: Area of Body*	Unproductive thoughts concerning creation.
Bites	Ignoring what is in the physical existence.
animal	Fear.
insect	Self pity or Self righteousness. This creates a stimulation of certain chemicals in the body causing it to be attractive to insects. These chemicals produced by the endocrine system include seratonin and adrenaline. Whether the cause is self pity or self righteousness depends upon the extent of the victimization in the attitudes.
Blackheads	Suppression of identity.
Bladder Problems	Refusal to release guilt and blame.

Remedy *Suggestions for Improvement*	*Personal Notes* *& Observations*
The universe is abundant. There is enough substance to fulfill your needs.	
Stop believing you can't fulfill desires for whatever reason. You can. Blaming others is just a cover up for your own feelings of inadequacy. You can build Self security and confidence by acting each day on your desires. No matter how small, the steps add up over time to create larger than life successes.	
Give freely and learn from love. State to your Self: "I came into this life to offer love."	
Direct the full, undivided attention to each experience in the environment, to the small and to the large.	
Always imagine desires, not fears.	
Understand how to cause growthful change.	
Communicate, talk and listen to what you have to say. Separate the productive from the unproductive. Retain the productive.	
You can't change the past, so place your attention on learning from the past and being productive in the present. Create the future you desire.	

Problem *Physical Disorder*	**Cause** *Mental Attitude Disorder*
Cancer of Bladder	Holding onto old ideas and hating Self for what has not been resolved. Refusing to release Self blame for unfulfilled desires and hating Self for it.
Bleeding (excessive)	Difficulty in building permanent understanding resulting in leaving lessons of life incomplete. Attachment to pain of injury.
Bleeding Gums	Neglect of Self.
Blindness *see: Eyes*	
Blisters	Refusing to admit where one is, resulting in a lack of respect for the body.
Blood Disorders	Attitude of Self weakness in responding to life and learning. Imaging the Self as being mentally weak or incapable.
Blood Pressure	Need to live up to one's own standards or expectations of what and who one can imagine becoming.
high	Expectations that are not being lived up to whether these are one's own or expectations of others. Being responsible for others.
low	Expectations of Self that one continually denies or refuses to admit. Listlessness or depression.

Remedy *Suggestions for Improvement*	*Personal Notes* *& Observations*
Use will power to direct the attention to the present. Find something you enjoy and love doing and immerse your Self in it even if it means making radical changes in your life.	
Recognize you have value and are a valuable human being. You are worth gaining value, learning, and growth in your experiences.	
Respect your Self. Start each day by doing something good for your Self.	
Admit your stage of learning. Consider, it is exciting to learn something new. "It is okay if I don't know everything. This means I can learn new lessons of life."	
Imagine accomplishing more than you ever have. Each day do something new that requires a little bit of courage.	
It is not your resonsibility to live for others. You are capable of fulfilling your own life and you need to, for this is the way you will aid the most people.	
You have the right and duty to have high expectations of Self. Communicate these to others and listen to their ideas and suggestions.	
Depression appears because you have denied the desires of Self. There needs to be action taken on your wants and needs. Admit who you are and that you are capable of much more than you have heretofore allowed your Self.	

Problem *Physical Disorder*	**Cause** *Mental Attitude Disorder*
Blood Problems see: *Leukemia, Anemia*	
clotting (lack of)	Thinking of Self as incapable of responding to the environment in order to build permanent learning.
clotting (excessive)	Closing Self off rather than using the ideas of Self for permanent understanding.
Body Odor (excessive)	Disgust or disdain held for Self.
Boils see: *Skin Disorders*	No communication to understand the thoughts that are being forced.
Bone(s) see: *Skeleton*	Thinking of Self as too old to learn or it is too late to cause change.
weakness	Believing there is no room for flexibility in the life or that there is no capability to create your desires.
Bone Marrow	Need to create a purpose for living. Refusal to live. Need to accept responsibility for creating the life as it is.
Bone Problems see: *Osteoporosis*	
breaks/fractures	Withdrawal of attention from the physical experience. Refusal to face facts in the physical life.

Remedy *Suggestions for Improvement*	*Personal Notes & Observations*
Begin to image Self as strong and willful.	
You lose nothing by listening. So be willing to listen to others.	
Give to others and give to Self. Practice love. Do things with your life that begin to aid you in liking your Self.	
Power comes from using and applying both the aggressive and receptive principles. Without communication to hear your own thoughts and those of others, there is little alteration of the ways that have not worked in the past. Initiate the new.	
Today influences the future, not the past. The effort put forth today does have an effect. There is always time to learn as long as you are willing.	
Begin to create stability in the life by creating mobility. Do something you have never done before. What have you been putting off for years?	
Building a purpose for living begins with creating a purpose for each activity performed. A purpose is a personal benefit.	
Each experience is useful for learning whether pleasant or unpleasant. It is through learning from experience that we are propelled to the next higher level of happiness and fulfillment.	

Problem *Physical Disorder*	**Cause** *Mental Attitude Disorder*
deformity	Hesitancy regarding the goals and purposes that have been set. Attachment to an idea that is no longer productive.
Bowels	Holding onto the past. Habitual thinking and actions.
Brain	Misuse or incomplete use of the thinking process. Scattered attention or incomplete use of the attention or imagination.
neurons	Scattering of attention.
axons	Difficulty in receiving impressions or perceptions.
dendrites	Difficulty in communicating perceptions.
synapses	Turning away from information. Often this is the result of drug usage.
pineal gland	Turning away from true Self.
cerebellum	Misuse of memory.

Remedy *Suggestions for Improvement*	*Personal Notes* *& Observations*
Set a goal for each day and accomplish it. Structure your life. Include flexibility within the structure.	
You can't change the past. You can change the present in order to create the future you desire. Begin now to change your Self. Make an improvement everyday. Be willing to admit when you are wrong or have made a mistake.	
Practice undivided attention for ten minutes each day on the object of your choice. For example, the tip of your finger, a candle flame, a pencil, or a blade of grass. Use your enhanced concentration throughout the day.	
Same as above. Remember to place your attention where the greatest learning is. Choose where you will place your attention. Do not allow your environment to determine the site of your attention.	
The true Self is the inner you. The real Self knows only forward motion, forward learning and growth. Identify with moving forward in life. Have an open mind to new learning and new opportunities.	
The true use of reasoning is to realize, "I created my Self and my life the way I am and it is. The cause of my life and situations begins with my thoughts."	

Problem *Physical Disorder*	**Cause** *Mental Attitude Disorder*
pituitary gland	Refusing to receive and interpret perceptions accurately.
hypothalamus	Identifying the Self as physical only. Refusing to admit the permanent understanding or permanent memory of Self.
thalamus	Doubt concerning the identity. Difficulty in understanding or embracing maturity in the Self. Confusion in thinking due to refusal to receive new information.
tumor (malignant)	Having received information where there is hatred of the information that has been received.
tumor (benign)	Feeling pressured or overwhelmed by information that has been received. Strong thoughts not brought to full awareness. Stubbornness, refusal to learn and resenting the learning process.
Breast Problems (female)	Holding onto old identity as a female.
cysts, lumps	Resentment or resistance to using the feminine expression.
Breathing Problems *see: Asphyxiating Attacks, Hyperventilation*	Fear or denial of the desires of Self. Believing other people are getting in the way of you fulfilling your real desires.

Remedy *Suggestions for Improvement*	*Personal Notes* *& Observations*
When listening with the senses, keep an open mind. Do not allow preconceived pictures to cloud perceptions.	
The physical body is your vehicle that you entered at the beginning of this lifetime and will leave at the end. The real you uses the vehicle to learn. You are not the vehicle.	
Practice meditation, concentration, and dream interpretation. You will come to know Self.	
Start liking your Self. Investigate your past and discover the times you did something that hurt another. Think of the times as a young child when you said or did something that hurt your parents, peers, or siblings. Forgive yourself.	
Any thought created is worthy of attention. Pay attention to your thoughts. The ones you don't like, that are unproductive, change.	
Realize we choose to be male or female for the learning the different vehicles (bodies) provide. Respect the choice you made to be female this lifetime. Identify the quality of receptivity and practice it.	
Begin by fulfilling some very small desire each day that you have been putting off.	

Problem *Physical Disorder*	**Cause** *Mental Attitude Disorder*
Bright's Disease see: *Nephritis*	
Bronchitis see: *Respiratory Ailments*	Thinking the desires of Self are not being fulfilled and blaming others for this.
Bruises	Oversensitivity in thinking one is always being injured by others emotionally.
Bulimia	Resenting the idea of control. Attention is directed towards pleasing others. Experiences created for the Self are interpreted according to how this will look or please someone else rather than being used for the learning of the Self. Since attention is focused on pleasing others, there is never the idea of Self having control. Desire to have what you want, when you want it regardless of consequences.
Bunions	Force occurring rather than exercising will power. Holding onto past ways of thinking.
Burns	Scattering of attention.
Bursitis see: *Area of Body*	Activity associated with area of body affected.
Buttocks see: *Systems of the Body*	Apprehension or some type of fear.
Callouses	Rigidity in thinking in terms of seeing only one way, rather than many different options thus causing energy blockage.

Remedy *Suggestions for Improvement*	*Personal Notes* *& Observations*
No one can fulfill your desires but you. Others may aid you when you communicate clearly. Practice communication, expressing both verbally and emotionally in a loving manner.	
The best attention is the attention you give your Self. Respect the space you occupy and the space other people and objects occupy.	
Control begins with having a clear mental image of who you want to be, how you want to express, and what you want to learn. Others cannot help you achieve your desires unless you know clearly what it is you desire.	
Will power is a series of unceasing steps toward a goal. Determination is utilized to make the ideal become reality.	
Practice concentration. The benefit is you experience more of reality.	
There is a proper tool for every job. Use the proper tool.	
Focus on desires.	
Produce learning in areas of your life you have not yet explored.	

Problem *Physical Disorder*	**Cause** *Mental Attitude Disorder*
Cancer	Hatred of Self.
Candida *see: Thrush, Yeast Infections, Ringworm*	
Canker Sores	Insecurity in expressing thoughts.
Car Sickness *see: Motion Sickness*	
Carbuncle *see: Boils*	
Carpal-tunnel Syndrome *see: wrist*	
Cataracts	Not wanting to see what the future holds in store.
Cellulite	Need for forward motion in the thinking process.
Cerebral Palsy *see: Palsy*	Blaming Self for mistakes and refusing to cause action as a form of correction.

Remedy *Suggestions for Improvement*	*Personal Notes & Observations*
Forgive your Self. Love your Self. Whatever has occurred in the past, you can be a productive and valuable individual today. People are not your enemy. The world is not the enemy. You are not the enemy. Care for others and love your Self.	
The only person that can really approve of you is you. At the end of this life, you will look back and decide if it has been productive and if you have accomplished what you desire. Therefore at the end of each day, examine and review that day to discover opportunities you could have used to communicate with others.	
Create your future with awareness by writing on paper what it is you desire to do with your life, what you want to create. Immediately begin creating action to fulfill this plan.	
Ask your Self this question, "What will produce more in my life than what I am presently accomplishing?" Imagine your Self being more than you presently are. Take steps toward your visualized thought image.	
The past is over. You cannot change it. However, you are capable of adjusting and adapting now, in the present. Start where you are. Cause motion where you can and reach for a little more each day.	

Problem *Physical Disorder*	**Cause** *Mental Attitude Disorder*
Cerebrovascular Accident *see: Stroke*	
Cheating	Worthlessness.
Childhood Diseases	
Congenital	Karma accepted to be fulfilled when choosing the parents.
2 - 6 years of age	Parental attitudes.
Chills *see: Endocrine System*	Holding back on responding. Difficulties with change or transformation of energies. Physically, imbalances within the endocrine system.
Cholesterol	
high	Lack of cooperation in terms of understanding responsibility and lack of usefulness in terms of existence.
arteriosclerosis	Living for others.
Chronic Disease or Illness	Pessimism. Desire for attention or false sense of importance. Thinking you have no ability to change Self or environment.
Chronic Liars	Thinking the ideas of Self have no worth.
Circulation **vascular/arterial systems**	Difficulty in understanding responsibility.

Remedy *Suggestions for Improvement*	*Personal Notes & Observations*
Create an honest assessment of Self worth.	
See specific illness and utilize suggestions.	
See area of body and disease.	
Create a balance within your Self. Are you too passive, letting the world pass you by or are you just the opposite, a bully? Instead be receptive and aggressive. Be a risk-taker.	
Slow your thoughts. Observe them. Choose productive thoughts, reject nonproductive thoughts. Respond to the positive.	
Investigate all jobs, occupations, avocations, hobbies. Question friends about what they do until you find something you enjoy doing for you. Make it work.	
Earn attention from others by creating success. Love Self, and others will find it much easier to love you.	
Each day make a statement of worth to another and also one to your Self. You can do this.	
The ability to respond and create your desires is freedom to fulfill desires. Do not confuse this with burden which is the refusal to imagine and act upon what you want in life.	

Problem *Physical Disorder*	**Cause** *Mental Attitude Disorder*
Cold Sores (Fever Blisters) *see: Herpes Simplex*	Hesitation in the expression.
Colds *see: Respiratory Ailments*	Indecision.
Colic	Emotion that is being absorbed without discrimination, primarily fear.
Colon *see: Intestines, Mucous Colon, Spastic Colon*	Holding onto the past.
Colitis	Holding onto failures and mistakes of the past and being angry about them. Blame.
Impacted Colon	Need to release blame.
Coma	Withdrawal of attention from the physical but has yet to be an assessment of what was learned. Indecision in regards to where the learning will take place next.
Congestion *see: Bronchitis, Colds, Influenza*	Feeling of imprisonment.
Conjunctivitis *see: Pink Eye*	

Remedy *Suggestions for Improvement*	*Personal Notes* *& Observations*
Practice saying what is on your mind and most importantly learn from your statements so you do not need to make it again.	
Make ten decisions each day that will produce forward motion in life. You can't make a decision not to do something. A decision is only a decision when there is action to produce motion.	
Practice undivided attention. Parents need to think productive and constructive thoughts and follow them with happy, joyous emotions.	
Change physical thinking to mental thinking. You only fail when you refuse to learn from the experience. If you learn, you will out-perform your previous endeavors.	
Prove to your Self, in the present, that you can still fulfill your desires.	
Blame stops release which stops your life. Begin to live now. Make something happen.	
Need to give undivided attention to the thoughts and who is behind the thoughts. Decide if you can still use this lifetime to learn and fulfill your purpose.	
Limitations are Self-created. Be decisive. Decide what you want and how to achieve it. Begin the process.	

Problem *Physical Disorder*	**Cause** *Mental Attitude Disorder*
Constipation	Holding onto the past. Procrastination resulting from holding onto the past.
Corns	Oversensitivity.
Coronary Thrombosis *see: Heart Attack*	
Coughs *see: Respiratory Ailments*	Blaming others for difficulty in fulfilling desires.
Cramps	Force. Pretending Self to be different from the present state of awareness.
Abdominal Cramps	Difficulties in receiving. Worry or anxiety concerning one's ability to respond to present conditions.
Croup *see: Bronchitis*	Desire for attention from others, particularly those in authority.
Cruelty *see: maliciousness*	
Crying (excessive)	Result of thoughts that are withheld. Therefore, there is the reaction in the emotions of pushing these thoughts to the surface.

Remedy *Suggestions for Improvement*	*Personal Notes* *& Observations*
The past isn't good enough anymore. You are worth more. The only place to build security is in the now. Security is caused by repeated success. Holding onto old worn-out attitudes causes slowing down of the learning process.	
There is nothing to lose by listening. Sticks and stones may break your bones but words can never harm you. Use the words that make sense and paint a picture of activity that will produce for you.	
When all else fails, change. Blaming others will produce no-thing for you.	
You have nothing to lose by being honest. Express your Self. Make your words match your thoughts. This is the only way you will know where you are in your awareness.	
Practice meditation every day for 15 minutes to an hour. Meditation is a receptive state called expectant non-action. Be receptive for the answer to your prayers or desires.	
Give love to others and they will love you. Parents need to give lots of love to children so the child knows he is loved.	
Share and give your thoughts and feelings to others. Listen to your Self so you may learn from your communication.	

Problem *Physical Disorder*	**Cause** *Mental Attitude Disorder*
Cushing's Disease see: *Adrenal Problems*	Imagining the Self to be the child when there is the need for maturity in Self.
Cuts see: *Injuries, Wounds*	Scattering of one's attention.
Cyst(s)	Unexpressed thoughts. Resentment.
Breast see: *Breast Problems*	Resentment of the feminine expression.
Cystic Fibrosis	Indecision concerning a goal or purpose for living. Passivity in causing a direction in life. No desires for life or nothing to give to life.
Deafness	Refusing to hear the truth.
Death	Withdrawing the attention from the physical existence.
Despair	Placing attention on imagined failures.
Dementia see: *Alzheimer's Disease, Senility*	Refusal to face physical realities or to discriminate what is physical from what is mental.
Depression	All of the attention on what is not had for the Self without creating goals or desires. Suppression of goals and desires.

Remedy *Suggestions for Improvement*	*Personal Notes* *& Observations*
Do something productive each day. Expand your horizons.	
Respect your Self enough to give your whole attention to whatever you do.	
Since you are valuable and important, your thoughts are important.	
Make a list of all the benefits of being female.	
You chose to incarn, to be in the physical and in a physical body, so get on with discovering your purpose in this lifetime by creating a purpose for living each day.	
The truth hurts for a little while, but the truth will set you free. Lies, dishonesty, and ignorance keep you in pain for a long time. Truth adds to and does not take away from.	
Ask your Self this question: "Have I done everything I came into this life to do?"	
Imagine farther into the future than has been imaged before.	
Find someone or something you love and give it your love, kindness, and attention.	
A not is no-thing. To produce something start with what you have. Make a list of the resources you have available including your physical possessions and your mental qualities and abilities. Now apply them toward achieving desires.	

Problem *Physical Disorder*	**Cause** *Mental Attitude Disorder*
Diabetes *see: Pancreas*	Refusing to give. Takes the form of deliberately withholding Self from others. Fear of never being able to have enough. Thinking Self does not have enough to give, therefore being stingy with how one gives.
Diarrhea	Thinking time is running out so wanting to get things over with rather than receiving and using what is available.
Digestive System	Refusal to embrace situations occurring in life. Difficulty in using experiences of life to gain knowledge of Self.
Diverticulitis	Holding onto old ideas from the past and allowing these thoughts to create anger in Self. Feeling trapped by the environment.
Diverticulosis	Holding onto old ideas from the past. Feeling trapped by the environment.
Dizziness (Vertigo)	Refusal to hear the inner Self or the thoughts of Self.
Doubt	Lack of Self worth.
Drug Addictions	Escape from physical reality or from facing facts.

Remedy *Suggestions for Improvement*	*Personal Notes* *& Observations*
Be courageous. You can't hide your Self forever, and fear is a limitation. Bring the real you out where others can see you. You may find you are a pretty valuable person.	
Stand in front of a mirror ten minutes each day and gaze at the reflection of your Self. Look at the face and head. Get to know and appreciate who you are.	
Ask your Self this question ten times each day, "What did I learn from the experience I just had?" This learning entails adding to your personality productively. It means you use each experience to improve your Self and make your Self a better person. What did you learn?	
By causing success in the present you won't have time to dwell on the past. Your anger was caused by your inability or unwillingness to control situations that occurred in the past. This does not have to be so in the present.	
Prove to your Self that you can still fulfill your desires.	
Practice concentration every day and when proficiency has been gained begin practicing meditation which is expectant listening to the inner Self.	
Practice causing fulfillment of desires.	
Find or cause a reason for living. Love something or someone who will return your love.	

Problem *Physical Disorder*	**Cause** *Mental Attitude Disorder*
Dysentery	Blaming the self for conditions that are not desirable. Idea of Self being weak and creating susceptibility in the body.
Dyslexia	Scattered attention occurring when one believes they are not capable of receiving what is available.
Ear(s)	Need to listen to Self. Lost in the thoughts of Self due to thinking others will not listen to ideas of Self. Mental hearing is needed.
Earache	Refusal to hear inner Self.
Eczema see: *Digestive/ Eliminatory Systems*	Holding onto old outworn ideas about Self as a way of hiding. Believing ideas of Self are unworthy thus restricting their expression.
Edema see: *Holding Fluids, Swelling*	Self righteousness. Holding onto old ideas from the past and feeling sorry for yourself.
Elbow see: *Joints, Arms*	
arthritis	Restriction caused by lack of purpose
injuries	Scattering of attention.

Remedy *Suggestions for Improvement*	*Personal Notes* *& Observations*
You are only weak when you refuse to set goals and act on them.	
Practice concentration exercises causing your attention to be in one place at a time. Discipline your imagination. The difference in scattered attention causing dyslexia or abrasions is with dyslexia the imagination jumps ahead; with abrasions the attention is kept in the past.	
Practice meditation and dream interpretation.	
Meditate for a minimum of 15 minutes each day.	
You can't hide from your Self. Find a way each day to make your Self a better person.	
Nobody is ever always right and nobody is ever always wrong. Appreciate your successes, however small, and learn from your mistakes so they won't be failures.	
Examine critically all preconceived notions and ideas. Write them out on paper. Which ones need adjustment and expanding upon? If you think the same way you did one year ago, you are not growing.	
Practice a concentration exercise ten minutes per day. Create a purpose for everything you do, thus aligning will and desire.	

Problem *Physical Disorder*	**Cause** *Mental Attitude Disorder*
Emphysema	Blaming Self or others for the unfulfillment of desires and for the restriction placed upon Self.
Encephalitis	Generalized indecision over whether one wants to use the body this lifetime. Withdrawal from life experiences.
Endocrine System	Difficulties with change in regards to the transformation of energies. It is linked to creative ability and the transforming of substance from one form of expression to another. Holding back on the response when a course of action has already been determined.
Endometriosis	Destroying femininity. Resenting the feminine expression, particularly the idea of powerlessness.
Epilepsy	Desire not to grow up. Refusing to face and learn from conditions present. Emotional overload.
Epstein-Barr Virus	Listlessness. Purposelessness of existence. Need for action on own desires.
Esophagus	Difficulty in receiving information.

Remedy *Suggestions for Improvement*	*Personal Notes* *& Observations*
Decide what you want and go after it. Make sure your desire benefits your Self and aids others. If you need to form new friendships, do so. A friend is not a friend if they try to hold you back in your learning and growth.	
You are in the physical and inhabiting a physical body for the purpose of learning. On paper, list ten reasons why you hate life, ten reasons why you are afraid of life, ten reasons why life can have meaning and value.	
Use courage in facing and challenging those areas of your life that you have been hiding from. Accept the belief into yourself that it is possible for you to create your fondest desires.	
You are beautiful. Write down ten ways you are a valuable person. Be good to your Self. Buy your Self some new clothes. Take that trip you have been wanting to take.	
Realize the fun begins when you grow up. You have much more freedom because you are able to respond to desires.	
Write out a Ten Most Wanted list. Number one on the list will be your most wanted desire. Number two will be your second greatest desire and so on down to number ten. Read this several times each day.	
Observe how the senses work. They are all receiving stations. No learning occurs without receiving.	

Problem *Physical Disorder*	**Cause** *Mental Attitude Disorder*
Eye Problems	Difficulties with mental perception. Need to make a decision concerning imagined goals.
Eyelids not opening after awakening	Attitude of rejection of the physical experience. Need to make a decision concerning imagined goals.
astigmatism	Distorted perception.
cataracts	Refusal to see the future clearly. Thinking of Self as too old to add anything to the mental vision, imagination, and perception.
exotropia	Difficulties in accurately perceiving what is within the environment or what is within the Self or both.
farsighted	Denial of the imagination.
keratitis	Refusing to face or perceive the present.
glaucoma	Clouding of one's perception from refusing to receive new ideas.

Remedy *Suggestions for Improvement*	*Personal Notes* *& Observations*
Cause the first step towards your visualized goals, no matter how small. Through the accomplishment of your first step, you will discover the second step. *Create a purpose or personal benefit for one activity a day, then expand it to two, and then to three. Next, create a purpose for everything you do.* *Do not allow preconceived notions to get in the way of accurately examining the present. View each experience as a totally new one. Do not prejudice your Self. Give learning a chance.* *Set goals for Self. Image them clearly. Act on them and you will see the future clearly. Practice directing undivided attention to each sense, one at a time. Next practice giving undivided attention to everyone you talk to and in each situation.* *Walk down a street, look to the right for ten seconds, turn your head forward and describe what you perceived in detail. Practice this until you can accurately describe what is in your environment.* *Practice gazing at your Self ten minutes each day in a mirror.* *Some of my best students who have changed the most were over 70 years old. It is never too late to grow if you will imagine and will it to be so.* *Practice listening. Receive the whole picture the other is presenting. Only after you have heard the whole picture, only then, start thinking.*	

Problem *Physical Disorder*	**Cause** *Mental Attitude Disorder*
nearsighted	Vagueness in creating goals.
temporary blindness	Denial of imagination.
walleyed *(see: Muscular Weakness, Nervous System*	Imagined goals or ideas that conflict with each other.
Face see: *Eliminatory System*	Hiding one's identity. Creating a false identity.
Failure	Lack of imagination.
Fainting	Refusing to learn.
Fat see: *Overweight*	
arms	Defensiveness.
belly	Protecting the Self from others.
hips	Misuse of the creative energy.
thighs	Difficulties in causing forward mental motion in Self.

Remedy *Suggestions for Improvement*	*Personal Notes* *& Observations*
Create a Ten Most Wanted list, using it each day. Set hourly, daily, weekly, monthly, yearly, and lifetime goals.	
Close your eyes and describe the clothes you are wearing or the car you drive. This is proof of your ability to visualize.	
Place your learning and growth as top priority. Then fit all goals and desires in relationship to this.	
Examine the things you say and the words you use. Are they accurately describing the thoughts you have? They must if you are to gain Self knowledge and improve Self.	
Imagine the condition desired.	
You gain no security in halting growth. Security comes from the repeated success of growth and learning. Begin now.	
Speak what is on your mind, with love.	
Words and thoughts will not harm you as long as you choose your own thoughts.	
Imagine a goal or desire and work towards it each day.	
Decide what you desire to learn next and seek out sources of this learning in your environment.	

Problem *Physical Disorder*	**Cause** *Mental Attitude Disorder*
Fatigue	Need to set goals. A contrast of thought between desire to create and doubt which results in limitations placed upon Self.
Fears	Need to direct the imagination productively.
Feet	Insecurities. When this attitude is present there is a way the body is held producing pressure on bones, muscles, and ligaments that reflects this insecurity. Neglect of giving one's attention to where one is at the present.
fallen arches	Thinking of Self as subservient.
Female Difficulties *see: Amenorrhea, Menstrual Problems, Vaginitis*	Difficulties in understanding the use of the feminine expression. Need to create in the life.
Fever *see: Toxins*	An effort made after a period of stagnancy or little learning to cause forward mental growth and expansion in the life.
Fever Blisters *see: Cold Sores, Herpes Simplex*	
Fibroid Tumors/Cysts *see: Tumors, Cysts*	

Remedy *Suggestions for Improvement*	*Personal Notes* *& Observations*
Set a small goal for your Self and accomplish it. Then create a slightly larger goal and accomplish this. If you need to place your Self in a new environment or for new friendships do so. Use the whole world to create your desires.	
Curiosity.	
Remember, security comes from repeated, mental success. Learn anew each and every day.	
Be the master of your life. You begin this process by outlining a series of goals and activities you desire to accomplish each day and appreciating each success. You may be crestfallen due to missing out on something you really desired in the past.	
Learn the value and power of receiving. Practice listening with all five senses.	
It is the small steps each day that add up to the big steps, the big accomplishments.	

Problem *Physical Disorder*	**Cause** *Mental Attitude Disorder*
Fingers	Scattering of attention. Neglect of a purpose for directing the attention.
Flatulence see: *Digestive Disorders*	Thinking that there will never be enough.
Flu see: *Influenza*	
Food Poisoning	Denial of Self.
Foolhardiness	Desiring to impress others.
Foot Problems	Need to give attention to mental foundation.
Fractures see: *Bone Disorders*	
Frigidity	Insecurity in responding when receptivity is required.
Fungus	Fearing invasion of Self by others. Irresponsibility in thinking. Mentally, an adolescent type of thinking that needs direction.
Furuncle see: *Boils*	
Gall Bladder	Trying to control others due to a fear of being controlled. Fear of being out of control. Envy. Manipulative quality.

Remedy *Suggestions for Improvement*	*Personal Notes* *& Observations*
Imagine a personal benefit for everything you do. Next, imagine benefitting others by adding to your Self.	
Reason with each experience to discover what can be learned that will aid in overcoming the limitations of the past.	
You are a unique, valuable person. Practice gazing at your face ten minutes a day in the mirror. Communicate your thoughts to others and listen.	
Understand the worth of your Self.	
Practice mental discipline.	
Create daily desires to fulfill and follow through upon them. Use will to conquer little steps to prepare for the large.	
Begin to appreciate experimentation and cause Self to reach for mental adulthood. Instead of building a wall up around yourself, a fort which will become your prison, build a warmth and lovingness that you share with others.	
Practice loving Self and loving where Self is within your own growth cycle, therefore, being able to respect other individuals and their choices.	

Problem *Physical Disorder*	**Cause** *Mental Attitude Disorder*
reduced functioning	Refusing to take control of one's own thoughts, emotions, and reasoning.
gallstones	Stubbornness in the thoughts creates attempts to force Self's way of thinking on others. Attempting to control others rather than controlling one's own thoughts.
Gangrene	Self destruction. Restriction of thoughts in the direction of forming and expressing understanding and truth.
Gas Pains (flatulence) see: *Digestive System, Intestines*	Hurrying.
Gastritis see: *Stomach Problems*	Scattered thinking in conjunction with information that is being accumulated, therefore new ideas are not easily digestible within the thinking processes. Worry or anger, especially when eating.
Genital Problems	Dislike or discomfort with the choices made in life relating to creativity. Misuse of the creative expression of power.
Genetic Code	Identity needs to be formed.

Remedy *Suggestions for Improvement*	*Personal Notes* *& Observations*
Set out to prove to your Self that you have value at the very core. Accept challenges and learn from the experience. You can be more and accomplish more than you thought possible, including self growth.	
Hold your attention on the desire that you personally desire to achieve each day. Use your own energy to make it happen.	
Cause thought to move more regularly in one direction. Be directed by your own desires.	
Take time to appreciate each moment to the fullest instead of rushing through it just to get it over with.	
Concentrate! Adopt the idea of being able to accomplish what is desired by slowing the mind to the point of listening to what is being offered. Give your full attention to the food you eat. What is the food's taste? Is it sweet, sour, salty, or bitter? What is the food's aroma? What is its texture, is it hot or cold?	
Become more familiar with the qualities of the masculine or feminine expression that have been chosen.	
Each day discover something about who you are. Observe your thoughts for ten minutes each day.	

Problem *Physical Disorder*	**Cause** *Mental Attitude Disorder*
DNA	Difficulties in how the identity is formed.
chromosomes	same
genes	same
RNA	Thoughts that are not responded to with action. Passivity in terms of directing thoughts.
Gingivitis	Neglect.
Gland(s) *see: Specific Gland*	Refusing to create.
Glandular Fever	Wanting to remove Self from situations due to lack of purpose in Self. Being angry about not fulfilling your true desires and blaming the environment.
Goiter *see: Thyroid*	Stubbornness in holding on to decisions made in the past that no longer apply to the present. Passivity in the use of will.
Gonorrhea *see: Venereal Disease*	Resentment of the sexual expression. Misuse of creativity. Destructiveness towards Self.
Gout	Regretting past understood experiences and learning. Guilt or regret, particularly revolving around irresponsibility.

Remedy *Suggestions for Improvement*	*Personal Notes & Observations*
Observe the thought of Self 15 minutes each day until you discover who is behind the thoughts.	
Identify wasted thought and energy each day. Eliminate waste from the life.	
Give your Self attention.	
Put two or more objects together each day in a way that is more productive than they were the day before.	
Activate purpose in your life. See how each activity toward a goal will add to your Self.	
Replace compulsive thinking with will and decision making. Have an open mind to hearing new ideas. Cause there to be more direction in the exchange of the giving and receiving cycle.	
Build respect for Self. Evaluate, see the worth, and use the value of Self and the learned experiences.	
Write out on a sheet of paper all the valuable activities of your life. Think about the many ways you have helped others. Appreciate the worth of what you have accomplished.	

Problem *Physical Disorder*	**Cause** *Mental Attitude Disorder*
Gray Hair	Thoughts of being pressured. Need to direct thoughts productively rather than constantly thinking compulsively.
Grinding Teeth	Difficulty releasing attention from concerns or problems.
Growths *see: Eliminatory System*	Difficulty in releasing information, habits, or doubts in Self .
Guilt	Placing the attention in the past on past mistakes.
Gum Problems *see: Digestive System*	Need to assimilate experiences into the Self.
Hair (falling out)	Refusal to follow through upon the thoughts. Self denial of pretending to be something you know your Self not to be.
Halitosis *see: Bad Breath*	Fear of learning stemming from a sense of worthlessness.
Hands	Need to develop and define Self's purpose.
Hatred	Removing attention from the desires of Self.

Remedy *Suggestions for Improvement*	*Personal Notes* *& Observations*
Choose the thoughts daily that are in alignment with your goals and desires. Hold your attention on productive thoughts.	
Read from a book you really enjoy for 30 minutes each night immediatly before going to bed. Choose a book haveing nothing to do with your troubles or problems of the day.	
Identify old ways. Admit specific ways of unproductive thinking that are continually dwelled upon then change them to productive thoughts and cause productivity with your life.	
Cause action in the present period of time.	
Each experience offers a valuable learning opportunity. Decide the quality or area of Self where you desire improvement and use your activity to do so.	
Share the real Self with others. You are a good person if you will let others get to know you. The Real you is valuable enough, you don't have to pretend to be something you are not.	
Behind every fear is a desire. Place your attention on those desires.	
What is the purpose? Write out how you would like to improve. What desires have yet to be fulfilled?	
Give attention to Self and create your desires.	

Problem *Physical Disorder*	**Cause** *Mental Attitude Disorder*
Hay Fever see: *Allergies*	Reaction and oversensitivity to the environment. Mentally distancing Self from the situation.
Headaches see: *Migraine Headaches*	Refusing to act on desires creating pressure on Self. Fighting needed change. Procrastination is often a factor.
Heart see: *Blood Disorder*	Misuse or misunderstanding of responsibility. Trying to compete with others in life when they have desires different from your own. Pretending to be content in an area but actually discontent due to not being where one aspires to be or where one thinks one should be.
heart attack	Stubbornness in refusal to admit that circumstances and conditions do not match within the thoughts and situation. Misunderstanding of responsibility as a burden. Fearing responsibility.
Heartburn see: *Peptic Ulcer, Stomach Problems, Ulcers*	Fear of not getting ahead. Difficulty in assimilating information. Placing attention on what the Self does not want to occur. Need to be aware of steps taken in the life. Need to assimilate experiences.
Hemorrhoids	Holding back on the expression of thought, then compensating reaction of forcing these thoughts at an unrelated or inopportune time.

Remedy *Suggestions for Improvement*	*Personal Notes* *& Observations*
Communicate the true thoughts, the true needs, and true desires of Self. Others will help you and be your friend.	
Respond to desires quickly. Allow no situation to get out of hand by postponing needed action.	
Display the Self in a way that is honest to the Self. Don't worry about whether your neighbor has a bigger house or a fancier house than you do, that is not what is important. What is important is that you decide what you want even if that is different from what everyone else wants. Live your life, not someone else's life.	
Set goals and direction for the Self to move forward. See above.	
Imagine desires being fulfilled. Communicate those desires to others.	
Share your thoughts with others for they deserve to learn of your ideas. You are a wonderful person and have much to offer the world. Next, initiate action on your ideas.	

Problem *Physical Disorder*	**Cause** *Mental Attitude Disorder*
Hepatitis see: *Liver Problems*	Despair. No reason to live. Cynicism concerning life ideals.
Hernia	Force. Restriction of creativity and mental desires of Self. Need to use wise judgement.
herniated disc	Ignoring conditions around the Self.
Herpes see: *Venereal Disease*	Guilt or insecurity concerning one's identity.
genital herpes	Guilt or insecurity in the sexual expression.
Herpes Simplex see: *Cold Sores*	Insecurity in the expression.
herpes labialis	Guilt and insecurity in the sexual expression.
Hiatal Hernia	Holding onto the past. Having the attention in the past, particularly on past mistakes. Information received is not processed in the thinking, it is related according to past ideas only.

Remedy *Suggestions for Improvement*	*Personal Notes* *& Observations*
It is time to decide what you really want to do with your life. What is the desire you have put off and attempted to ignore for years? Do it!	
Know your own limitations and each day continue to expand beyond them so you move beyond the old, outworn concepts of Self.	
Respect your body and your environment, giving them attention.	
Seek methods of discovering who you are, where you came from, and where you are going.	
Do your own research. Research human anatomy; male and female. Practice loving people.	
Practice being yourself when with others.	
Be honest in your relationships with others.	
Write down the major attributes of your mother and father, and your older brothers and sisters. Write down also anyone else you modeled yourself after. Look to see if you were taught limitations, negativity, or worthlessness by any of these people. Begin to change the attitudes you had adopted by replacing the limited thoughts with more expansive thoughts. Model yourself after some successful people.	

Problem *Physical Disorder*	**Cause** *Mental Attitude Disorder*
Hip Problems	Self denial, particularly of the creative expression.
Hives *see: Rash*	Holding back in the emotional expression.
Hodgkin's Disease	Fear of responsibility. Difficulty with identification of who the Self is in relationship to life.
Holding Fluids *see: Edema, Swelling*	Holding back on the thoughts of Self.
Hot Flashes	Thinking of Self as powerless or incapable of causing change and angry about this.
Huntington's Disease	Refusal to create purpose for living. Lack of emotional control. Refusal to reach out to the environment to experience and learn.
Hydrophobia	Fear of the unknown.
Hyperactivity	Scattered attention without awareness of the ability to direct the attention.
Hyperglycemia *see: Diabetes*	
Hypertension	Feeling overburdened and that life is too much to handle.

Remedy *Suggestions for Improvement*	*Personal Notes* *& Observations*
Spend ten minutes looking at yourself each day in the mirror. Love Self.	
Share your ideas with others using enthusiasm and excitement for life. It is worth living!	
Your responsibility to you is to learn and grow. It is through the process of growth that we discover who we are. Create ways to learn each day.	
Replace fear with desire. Behind every fear is a desire to mature and produce. On the left side of a sheet of paper, list your fears. Across from this on the right side write down the hidden desire.	
Eat one food each day that you normally do not eat. Cause yourself to enjoy that food.	
Give love to a pet. Spend time with nature. Smell the air. Feel the breeze. Relax and love being with nature.	
Practice creating desire to know.	
Practice concentrating on the tip of your finger for ten minutes each day, or you may use a candle flame.	
The ability to respond is a freedom and is never a burden. Remember your goal. Remember your purpose and life will never be a burden again. Love the present moment, the now.	

Problem *Physical Disorder*	**Cause** *Mental Attitude Disorder*
Hyperthyroidism *see: Goiter*	Making choices or decisions without thought or responsibility as to their consequences. Scattering of attention so there is not the completion of thoughts, therefore, will is directed rapidly and weakly for short terms in many directions diluting the will's effectiveness.
Hyperventilation	Fear from not having faced conditions.
Hypoglycemia *see: Pancreas, Diabetes*	Refusing to believe you have anything within Self of value or worth to offer or give another. Thinking of Self as weak and using this to manipulate others.
Hypothyroidism *see: Thyroid*	Mental laziness.
Ileitis (Crohn's Disease)	Blame. Passivity created when there is a lack of fulfilling desires and there is a giving up that is a form of defense. Anger at missing and not using opportunities in the past and present.
Ileocecal Valve	Idea that receiving something new is taking away from what has been built in the past. Scattering of attention causing ignorance of the present moment or the now due to the attention going to the past habitually. Need to cause peace in one's own thinking by appreciating what has been accomplished and where one wants to go in the future.
Impotence	Insecurity in responding when the aggressive quality is required.

Remedy *Suggestions for Improvement*	*Personal Notes & Observations*
Practice making decisions each day. Choose a different route to go to work rather than being habitual. Examine your life to discover all the habitual tendencies you practice daily. Replace them with decision making and will power.	
Stop procrastinating! Begin making decisions that put you in the driver's seat each day.	
If you think you have to resort to manipulation of others to have control of your life, then you really have very little ability to fulfill desires. Build mental strength by doing!	
Challenge yourself to imagine, to remember, to decide, and to reason. Build a strong will by developing a purpose for everything you do.	
The present is always better than the past when the imagination is used to initiate a building cycle.	
Make a list of your major accomplishments in life. Appreciate your achievement. Now draw up a future list of accomplishments based on your most heart felt desires.	
Ask your Self, "What is it I really want to say and do?" Stop waiting for others to give you instruction on what to do and start showing some individual initiative.	

Problem *Physical Disorder*	**Cause** *Mental Attitude Disorder*
Incontinence (loss of urinary control)	Withdrawal of attention from the physical body. Fear of maturing. Thinking of Self as powerless or out of control. Refusal to see any value in the past experiences.
Incurable	Refusal to live or no idea of how to cause change.
Indigestion	Attention being given to something other than what is presently in front of the Self.
Infection *see: Viral Infection*	Defensiveness, perceiving Self as weak or defenseless.
Inflammation	Suppressed anger. Overreaction to outer or inner environment due to defensiveness.
Influenza *see: Respiratory Ailments*	Indecision. Occurs when attention has been given to the thoughts and there is still the recognition by Self that there needs to be action taken and there is still procrastination.
Ingrown Toenail	Need for proper perspective in life. Primarily from physical causes.

Remedy *Suggestions for Improvement*	*Personal Notes & Observations*
Express ideas. Share wants, needs and aspirations. Accept with joy new opportunities for the freedom of leadership and ability to respond.	
Decide what you would really like to do if you had no restrictions. Now do something about it. Start with anything. Just do something. Doing something is always better than nothing for by doing something you have the opportunity to learn.	
Give your full attention to the food you are eating. What does the food look like, smell like, taste like, sound like, feel like? Give your full attention to the now.	
The real Self can never be destroyed so speak, act, and be from the Real you, then there is no need to defend your right to exist.	
Consider each situation as a totally new opportunity to learn. Then life is fun instead of something to be feared or angry about. Anger occurs from a reaction of feeling you have no control so visualize your goals and desires, moving toward them. Make your dependency be on Self first, then when you are dependable you will be able to depend upon others.	
Make ten decisions each day different from the decisions you would normally make and follow through on them.	
Give your body the respect it deserves. Take care of your body.	

Problem *Physical Disorder*	**Cause** *Mental Attitude Disorder*
Injuries see: *Cuts, Wounds*	Scattering of attention.
Insanity	Refusing to face reality in terms of separating what is physical from what is mental and being willing to cause and respond to learning in physical life.
Insomnia	Procrastination. Inability to release attention from conscious thoughts.
Intestines see: *Colon*	Holding onto the painful past and refusal to embrace and use the present. Holding onto or rejecting ideas whether past or present opinions.
Isles of Langerhans see: *Pancreas*	Selfishness. Dependency issues.
Itching see: *Skin and Toxins*	
"itis" see: *Inflammation*	Anger.
Jaundice see: *Liver Problems*	No purpose for living.
Jaw Problems see: *Skeletal System*	Mental and emotional tension. Need to follow through on ideas and release concerns of the day. Replaying memory scenes without resolving inner stress reactions.

Remedy *Suggestions for Improvement*	*Personal Notes* *& Observations*
If an action is worth doing, it is worthy of your attention.	
Ask yourself: "What do I want to do with my life and how can I find more purpose and meaning to life?" Begin the practice of meditation.	
Before you go to bed at night ask yourself this question, "Is there something I could have done today that I didn't?" If the answer is yes, then do it.	
Why live in the past? Now is the time to enjoy life. Now is the time to live life to the fullest. Once each day prove the limitation of something you were told as a child or earlier in your life. This you will use to expand beyond preconceived biases and limitations.	
Give to someone each day. Give something of your Self each day. Do something beneficial for someone each day.	
Respect your Self to begin causing what you want in your life each day without trampling over others.	
You need to decide to do what you want to do. Stop telling yourself why you can't have what you want and begin to find ways to prove to your Self you can have what you desire.	
If you openly share your ideas with others and put them into practice, then you will gain the flexibility to use other's ideas. You will find a freedom you have never experienced.	

Problem *Physical Disorder*	**Cause** *Mental Attitude Disorder*
Jealousy	Procrastinating on fulfilling one's desires.
Joints *see: Arthritis, Elbow, Knee*	Mental restriction.
Keratitis *see: Eye Problems*	Attachment to hurt. Blocking the perception of a particular thought.
Kidney Problems	Guilt and condemnation. Placing blame on Self for mistakes made rather than looking for and understanding the cause.
stones	same
Knee *see: Joints*	Restriction within the thinking.
Laryngitis	Holding back on what is desired to be said.
Left Side of Body *see: Area of Body*	
Leg(s) *see: Area of Leg*	
Leprosy	Self destruction. Fear of responsibility.

Remedy *Suggestions for Improvement*	*Personal Notes* *& Observations*
Cause action toward fulfillment of desires.	
Eliminate for six months from your life and vocabulary: "I can't, I won't, I shouldn't, I couldn't, and I haven't." Replace them with I can, I will, I want to, I am able.	
It is time to stop allowing old memory patterns to override the present experience. See situations for what they are and not what they used to be.	
The past cannot be changed, but the present, not the past, determines your future. Therefore, stop trying to live in the past. Begin now to create anything you desire. Love your Self.	
same	
Choose one limitation you have placed on your Self and overcome it.	
Are you afraid of being hurt if you say what you honesty think and see? If so, then remember to keep the other person's best interest in mind and communicating will be easier.	
The first thing to do is to convince your Self you are a worthwhile individual and you do have something valuable to contribute to your fellow man.	

Problem *Physical Disorder*	**Cause** *Mental Attitude Disorder*
Leukemia	Resentment revolving around imagined injustices creating defensiveness. Extreme rejection of ideas of responsibility for life.
Leukorrhea *see: Female Problems*	Weakness seen within Self and hating Self for this weakness particularly in regards to using the receptive side of creation. Feeling of helplessness.
Limbic System	Superficiality of the emotions.
Liver *see: Hepatitis, Jaundice*	Attitude of worthlessness leads to feeling useless. Difficulties in understanding or creating purpose in life. Need to build Self respect.
Lockjaw *see: Tetanus*	Neglect of one's own needs. Fear of foreign influences.
Low Energy Level	Need to cause there to be more activity mentally.
Lou Gehrig's Disease *see: Amyotrophic Lateral Sclerosis*	
Lump in Throat	Refusal to use the will to express the thoughts.
Lump in Breast	Difficulty in understanding the quality of nurturing.

Remedy *Suggestions for Improvement*	*Personal Notes & Observations*
This extreme resentment causes you to think you have to defend yourself constantly against the whole world. Change this. Learn to love your Self and to give love to all you come into contact with.	
Read books about famous women of the past and present. Discover and practice the power of creativity.	
Be your Self. Express your thoughts honestly but learn from your expression so you do not need to repeat the unproductive.	
Begin respecting your Self. You are an important individual. Through practicing purpose each day, we can see progress in our lives. This creates Self respect and a purpose for living.	
Basic needs are food, shelter, and clothing. Other needs are friendship and communication. Higher needs are for learning, growth, awareness, and self development.	
Create a purpose for life. Develop a personal benefit for everything you do.	
Do something to complete that which has been imagined.	
Aid others to learn and grow. Teaching would be an excellent vehicle.	

Problem *Physical Disorder*	**Cause** *Mental Attitude Disorder*
Lung *see: Pneumonia*	Thinking one's desires will not be fulfilled and blaming others for this. Feeling a loss of freedom of expression. Fearing the desires of Self will not be fulfilled.
Lupus	Bitterness from trying to manipulate others and not being able to do so. Insecurity in the belief in Self and one's ability to fulfill desires.
Lymphatic System	Defensiveness. Self pity. The idea of powerlessness to cause change. Self pity is a form of defensiveness as a way of denying desires.
lymph nodes	Defensiveness.
lymphatic cancer	Apathy taking over after cancer is already in the body. Apathy following hatred.
Malaria	Feeling overwhelmed by pressure and responsibility.
Maliciousness	Denying one's desires and then blaming others for the lack of fulfillment of your desires.
Mastitis *see: Breast Problems*	Rigidity in the thinking processes, particularly concerning femininity.
Melanoma	Distaste or disgust for the image one has of the Self.

Remedy *Suggestions for Improvement*	*Personal Notes* *& Observations*
Your life begins with your thoughts. Therefore decide what is truly desired in the life. Write the desires down in order of importance.	
Others do not give you happiness. Happiness begins with Self. Practice meditation each day to get in touch with the inner Self.	
Give so that you may create and fulfill your desires. Feeling sorry for yourself will not get you what you want. Creating clear mental images of needs and directing effort toward them will.	
Offensively, give to others without condition, freely. You control your environment by giving.	
You need to learn to love your Self and love life.	
Do your best each day. Tomorrow improve what you did today. Always look for and seek improvement.	
Give your Self permission to create and live your inner desires.	
Give, give, give from the depths of your being, for in giving the bonds of limitation are released.	
Imitate those you hold in high regard. Develop a type of expression of your personality that is beneficial to others.	

Problem *Physical Disorder*	**Cause** *Mental Attitude Disorder*
Melitis	Holding back on what there is to give of the identity. Feeling as if one has a worthless expression and being angry about this.
Memory Difficulties	Ignoring thoughts and emotions.
Menopause Problems	Reluctance to adjust to change and embrace the future in order for there to be mental maturing.
Menstrual Problems *see: Amenorrhea, Female Difficulties*	Misuse of or insecurity in use of the feminine expression.
cramps	Difficulty in receiving.
Migraine Headaches *see: Headaches*	Feeling pressured by factors that seem out of one's control.
Miscarriage	Indecision or doubt upon the part of the mother in regards to this one's identity as a mother.
Mononucleosis *see: Glandular Fever*	Indecision practiced over a long period of time regarding a particular issue or experience that is never resolved.
Morning Sickness	Hesitation or insecurity regarding change. Insecurity or second thoughts regarding pregnancy.

Remedy *Suggestions for Improvement*	*Personal Notes* *& Observations*
Give your thoughts, ideas, time, effort, and energy. Give your Self towards aiding others in leading a better life and you will prosper in return.	
Face the past and present with undivided attention. Examine your memories. Learn from them and release your attachment.	
If you use everything learned to this point in your life, then there is the capacity available to improve the quality of life.	
The power of receptivity beings with listening. Begin!	
Give, give, give! So you may receive, receive, receive. Relax, slow down, cooperate with others.	
Ask your Self ,"What is it I really want to do, to say, to be?" Move in this direction.	
Practice meditation to discover who you are. Practice concentration to discover your thoughts. Discover the benefits and learning from motherhood, if motherhood is your desire.	
Each of us has free will. We have love, caring, communication, the ability to give and receive, and the ability to imagine. Make small decisions daily that are different from habitual actions of the present. This will lead to unexpected, beneficial results.	
Be in the present now. You cannot live in the future. You can create your future by being productive in the eternal now.	

Problem *Physical Disorder*	**Cause** *Mental Attitude Disorder*
Motion sickness (car, sea, air sickness)	Having one's attention in the future rather than in the present.
Mouth Problems	Difficulty with expressing one's thoughts.
Mucous Colon *see: Colitis, Colon, Intestines, Spastic Colitis*	Need to release ideas of the past.
Multiple Sclerosis	Desire to run from learning. Placing blame or refusing to be responsible for conditions and circumstances in the life.
Muscles	Straining or forcing, due to holding on to unproductive thoughts, therefore not efficient use of energies. Need to understand how the mind causes the vehicle (body) to function. Retarding of actions on mental creations. Refusal to be honest with Self in regards to one's strength or capacity and one's capacity to cause motion and change.
biceps	Identifying with weakness, straining or forcing regarding the idea one holds of strength when one is afraid the Self will not be strong enough.
deltoids	Pretending to be something other than what one is. Need to be honest with Self image. Trying to prove Self physically.
quadriceps	Using force rather than power to try to please others. A showing off attitude producing strain on this area in the actions performed.

Remedy *Suggestions for Improvement*	*Personal Notes* *& Observations*
Look for something of interest in your environment. Practice undivided attention. Love your life so you will be here now.	
Go ahead, say what is on your mind for it is not worth getting sick over.	
Practice loving your Self in order to forgive your Self for the past that no longer exists.	
You can't escape from learning, so begin to love life and love your Self.	
Begin practice of meditation, concentration, memory enhancement, dream interpretation, visualization, and healing as tools for understanding the mind. Begin to create your imagined desires.	
Remember, real power begins with the mind. For any lasting creation to occur, productive and clear thoughts must be present. Visualize your desires each day upon arising.	
The fake you is never as good as the real you. So be the real you. You can only get better!	
When one procrastinates until the last possible moment, there tends to be a lot of energy expended to change events once they are already set in place. Respect others.	

Problem *Physical Disorder*	**Cause** *Mental Attitude Disorder*
sterno-mastoid	Identifying with weakness but pretending strength on the outside. Emotional restriction therefore forcing the expression of emotion.
trapezius	Tension regarding the inner desires and the desire to please others. Force in terms of forward motion.
triceps	Using force rather than power. Doing beyond one's capability.
Muscular Dystrophy	Refusal to use the will to cause motion in life.
Muscular Tension	Unexpressed thoughts.
Myocardial Infarction see: *Heart Attack*	Misuse of responsibility.
Myopia see: *Eye Problems*	Attention too far in the future without definition.
Nails	Need to give attention to purpose and using energy.
Nail Biting	Need to express and communicate purpose.
Narcolepsy	Denial of stimulation to learn. Desire to escape based upon information that is being received without the willingness to understand.

Remedy *Suggestions for Improvement*	*Personal Notes* *& Observations*
Admit who you are and the limit of your present abilities. Next begin to move beyond these limits. As long as you continue to lie or pretend, you cannot move forward for forward motion must be built on honesty.	
If you don't fulfill your desires you won't be happy, and therefore you will not aid others to happiness. Decide what it is that you want.	
Initiate steps to your goal, <u>each day</u>.	
Imagination leads to desire. Desires stimulate the ego to create forward motion by exercising the will.	
Say what is on your mind without attacking another. Say it with love and face your fears.	
Stop trying to keep up with your next door neighbor and start improving your life in the direction <u>you</u> really desire even when your desires are different from others.	
Love your Self and love the present. Find joy in the present experience.	
Respect food as nourishment for your body which is the vehicle for you, the soul or I AM.	
You can achieve what you imagined. Believe this and cause Self to prove the truth of it.	
Banish fear. Identify your worse fears. Now identify your greatest desires. Move on the desires, and the fears over time will vanish.	

Problem *Physical Disorder*	**Cause** *Mental Attitude Disorder*
Nausea	Anxiety concerning the present and too much attention given to future worries.
Nearsightedness *see: Eye Problems, Myopia*	Vagueness in the goals that relate to the distant future, seeing the future as very far off.
Neck (cervical spine)	Viewing responsibility as a burden. Need to use the imagination and will.
Neck Problems *see: Spinal Misalignments - special section, Stiff Neck)*	Need to use will.
Nephritis *see: Bright's Disease*	Condemnation of the Self for the past and holding on to anger about this. Waste, in terms of ways of thinking or choices that have not been productive, that are not released.
Nervous Breakdown	Shutting off mental attention in an attempt to avoid confronting situations present in the life.
Nervousness	Scattered attention.
Nervous System	Need to give attention to receiving and using information productively. Misuse of attention.
Neuralgia	Removal of attention from physical stimuli and reduction therefore in learning.
Nodules *see: Digestive System*	

Remedy *Suggestions for Improvement*	*Personal Notes* *& Observations*
Create the future by concentrating on being effective in the present.	
Write down all the steps it will take to achieve this year's goals, this decade's goals, and your lifetime goals. Each day fulfill a step.	
Respond, respond, respond. This is freedom.	
Tomorrow start off the day as if it were the beginning of a whole new life.	
Be totally open minded to new ideas, new ways of doing activity, and new ways of perceiving life.	
You can never escape from your Self, you can only put it off making your life painful. Anything you create, you can handle.	
Concentrate.	
Ten times each day, touch someone and describe out loud what the touch is like. Practice describing the flavors of foods.	
Watch a child under the age of seven for one hour a day for one month. Watch to see the joy the child experiences in new learning. Imitate the joy of the child until you can create it at will.	

Problem *Physical Disorder*	**Cause** *Mental Attitude Disorder*
Nose	
bleeds	Wanting to escape.
runny	Indecision or hesitation.
stuffy	Self pity.
Numbness	Withdrawing attention from what is present in the environment.
Osteomyelitis *see: Bone Problems*	Identification with weakness. Need to use structure to create instead of being angry because the structure isn't the way one wants it to be.
Osteoporosis *see: Bone Problems*	Thinking Self is no longer capable of changing or restructuring the life in order to grow and develop.
Ovaries	Difficulty in the use and power of the feminine expression. Misuse of the receptive expression.
Overweight *see: Fat*	Believing one needs to protect or defend the Self. Unfulfilled desires give rise to mistrust.
Pain	Denial of need to give attention.
Palsy *see: Paralysis, Parkinson's Disease*	Ignoring learning. Withdrawing the attention from the physical experiences.

Remedy
Suggestions for Improvement

Personal Notes
& Observations

Face yourself.

Make ten decisions each day different from the day before. Initiate action upon them.

Do something. Be productive. Try something new. Get a hobby that you love. Find something or someone to love.

The art of perception begins with giving full attention to where you are and what you are doing.

Write down all the things you can do. Write down all the skills, talents, abilities, and worthwhile knowledge you have. Create ways to use it.

Develop a new skill. Learn art or music. Start a new business. Develop something new, develop a new structure.

Practice meditation every day as a method of being receptive to the inner Self.

Trust Self. Act on desires of Self. Be who you are. Face your loneliness and share Self with others.

Create a purpose for everything you do then you will experience the pleasure of that activity instead of wanting to mentally ignore what you are doing.

At some point in your life you have decided that all life is painful, too painful for you to bear. This is a falsehood. Life is worth living. Concentrate on a fresh rose each day for ten

Problem *Physical Disorder*	**Cause** *Mental Attitude Disorder*
Pancreas	Desire to give and holding back on this. Fear of losing from giving. Attitude of Self righteousness which is selfishness. Conditionally giving and receiving. Jealousy.
Paralysis	Need to give attention to the desires of the inner Self. Accumulated passivity. Refusal to cause movement in forms of creative ability.
Parasites	Stealing from others.
Parathyroid	Insecurity in the identity. Refusal to cooperate with structure. Refusing to act on decisions that have been made to structure creativity. Associated with the action of the will and the need for subsequent movement to occur in form of structure.
Parkinson's Disease	Withdrawal from experience. A particular incident causes a shutting down or refusal to receive.
Pelvis (tilted) *see: Spinal Column and Skeleton*	Insecurity in the ability to create what one desires. Fear of not being able to excel or that time is running out.

Remedy *Suggestions for Improvement*	*Personal Notes & Observations*
minutes for one month. At the end of each day's ten minute effort, write down ten reasons why the rose is beautiful.	
Give freely of your Self. Have the courage to reveal the Real you. Give to ten people each day. Find a present for someone each week, a present that is very special and just exactly for that person.	
What do you really want from your existence? Deep down you want to give and receive love, caring, sharing, importance, value, respect, and worth. The first step is admitting these.	
What is stolen, you will lose. What you earn for the inner Self you will gain forever.	
Use your will to create a business, an invention, a healthier, stronger body, a house, etc. Learn to use structures already in existence.	
Create ways for pleasure in life to outweigh pain. Examine critically, clinically, and with love for Self and others, the particular experience. What frightened you, who or what are you afraid of? What would you desire to change about the past but can't. What can you do in the present to create a productive future?	
Do one thing you have never done before that is a challenge. Then continue creating challenges.	

Problem *Physical Disorder*	**Cause** *Mental Attitude Disorder*
Peptic Ulcer *see: Heartburn, Stomach Problems, Ulcers*	Attention placed on what one does not want to occur. Worry.
Periodonitis *see: Pyorrhea*	Neglect of nurturing one's Self.
Phlebitis	Rigidity in thinking. Confusion or irrationality in the thinking. Feeling angry because one has not responded to the inner desires of Self for a long time and now is trying to do so.
Piles	Force in the choices that are made. Forcing without responsibility.
Pimples *see: Blackheads, Whiteheads*	Insecurity in the identity and expression.
Pinkeye	Refusal to perceive opportunities for learning available. Hesitancy on action concerning what is perceived.
Pituitary Gland	Scattered attention or difficulties with using the thinking process productively. Refusing to visualize.
Pity (self pity)	Unfulfillment of desires and not admitting the responsibility of the Self in creating desires.
Plantar's Wart	Indecision.
Pneumonia *see: Lung Problems*	Fear of desires not being fulfilled. Repression of emotions. Hesitation or restriction in the words, actions, ideals that are held within Self so nothing occurs in terms of productive movement.

Remedy *Suggestions for Improvement*	*Personal Notes & Observations*
Imagine desires, not fears.	
Find ways to prove to Self that you are a valuable person.	
Examine your thoughts. Do something different each day. Begin to change or adjust any part of your life that is non-essential. Turn your life in a new, more productive direction.	
Instead of procrastinating, find joy in developing steps daily to fulfill goals.	
Speak, listen, and refine. You get better with practice. Communication is the key.	
Give your Self a chance. Ask: "What can I do that I had previously dismissed as impossible to accomplish?"	
Practice visualization, undivided attention, and memory exercises.	
Examine your ability to respond to and for the Self, then begin embracing life.	
Make ten decisions each day and act on them that same day.	
The only way to get over this fear is to act on desires of Self every day. Take a step. The reaction stems from oversensitivity to stimuli, particularly stimuli from other individuals which causes the reaction. The solution is to mentally create goals and desires for the Self	

Problem *Physical Disorder*	**Cause** *Mental Attitude Disorder*
Poisoning	Paranoia
Poison Ivy	Self pity or blame. Feeling sorry for the Self. Pity causes there to be a reduction in the strength of the immune system.
Poison Oak *see: Poison Ivy*	Self pity
Polio	Refusing to be responsible in action. Desire for escape. This produces a condition so there is not the physical means of escape.
Post-nasal Drip	Doubt or indecision.
Posture (poor) *see: Scoliosis*	Attitude of carrying others' burdens or responsibilities.
Premenstrual Syndrome (PMS)	Sluggishness in the creative thinking.
Proneness towards disease	Need for greater appreciation for Self and the expression of what can be created by the Self.
Prostate	Passivity. Difficulty in using the aggressive expression. Need to utilize the creative potential within Self. Dislike of sexual partner.

Remedy *Suggestions for Improvement*	*Personal Notes & Observations*
and everyday initiate one or more steps forward towards your most heart felt desires.	
Communicate.	
You have free will. You have used that free will to make decisions that created your life. Therefore, be excited for you can make decisions now that will create a much better, more exciting life.	
The best way to overcome Self pity is to immediately begin to do something productive.	
You are here. You have a physical body. Invent ingenious ways to create and be useful to your Self and others. You can be great!	
Make ten decisions each day, as described before.	
Everyone has free will. You must take care of your Self. If you continually ignore your desires you will experience unhappiness. It will be difficult in this condition to bring joy to others.	
Set monthly goals with steps to accomplish each day.	
Pain's purpose is to draw our attention to something that needs our attention. Be kind to your Self. Love your Self enough to be productive and grow.	
Initiate activity on a desire daily. Make that desire real and love it into existence.	

Problem *Physical Disorder*	**Cause** *Mental Attitude Disorder*
Psoriasis *see: Skin*	Holding back in the expression of thought.
Pubic Bone *see: Skeletal System*	Restriction in the creative expression.
Pyorrhea *see: Periodontitis*	Neglect of Self.
Rabies	Fear
Rash *see: Hives*	Oversensitivity in the thinking process. Hesitation or holding back in Self expression.
Rectum *see: Anus*	Holding onto the past, particularly blame.
Resentment	Sacrificing as a means of Self importance.
Reproductive System	Misunderstanding of the creative power.
Respiratory System *see: Bronchitis, Colds, Coughs, Influenza*	Mental restriction creating emotional repression from not fulfilling desires. Not verbalizing desires of Self due to thinking they have no value.
Revenge	Desire for understanding.

Remedy *Suggestions for Improvement*	*Personal Notes* *& Observations*
Thoughts are real. Thoughts exist. They must be acted upon and used. The unproductive thoughts are to be eliminated.	
Find two objects and put them together in such a manner as has never been done before.	
Love your Self into a greater existence.	
Look for the true desires. Place attention on these desires and act on them. The fears will be released.	
You are not bad. You are not a bad person. Everyone is not out to get you. Rather you have value and worth. Forgive, and love your Self and others.	
If you have made mistakes in the past that you will not release, then forgive your Self by giving to others.	
Others do not make you important, your quality of thinking and what you offer does. Understand the importance of the whole Self.	
Ask your Self this question at the beginning of each day, "How can I add to and improve on the factors, qualities, and conditions in my life?" Then proceed to do so.	
What excuse are you using for stopping your Self for no one else is stopping you. You may need to change jobs, locations, and/or people in your life, but you can have anything you desire.	
Cause understanding where there has been misunderstanding.	

Problem *Physical Disorder*	**Cause** *Mental Attitude Disorder*
Rheumatism	Mental prison that one creates in the thinking. Lack of mental forward motion.
Rheumatoid Arthritis	Feeling imprisoned by the thinking process. Identifying with limitations and being angry about this.
Rickets	Feeling out of control in regards to using structures.
Right side of body see: *Area of body*	
Ringworm	Need for balance of aggressive and receptive qualities within Self.
Root Canal see: *Teeth*	Neglect. Need for Self nurturing.
Round Shoulders see: *Shoulders, Spinal Curvature*	Holding on to ideas of failure. Feeling burdened.
Sagging Lines see: *Area of body*	Mental tension.
Scabies	Feeling overpowered by others and the environment. Shame.
Scarring	Attachment to pain or injury.

Remedy *Suggestions for Improvement*	*Personal Notes & Observations*
Why do you identify with limitation and lack? Instead, begin to create avenues to fulfill the desires of Self.	
Words describe the way one thinks. Listen to yourself and your words. Then listen to others particularly successful individuals. You will notice their words are different from yours and proceed from different mental pictures. Imitate theirs until you learn to produce success.	
Use every situation to the fullest. Never give up hope, for hope is a mental, imaged picture of how you want the world to be. Make efforts in the direction of your dreams.	
Talk and listen. Give and receive. Share and learn. Practice the opposites.	
Appreciate and respect your physical body.	
Burden and responsibility are two different experiences. Responsibility is freedom and always involves purpose. Burden is a chore or load that is contrary to desire and carried for someone or something outside of your Self.	
Remove attention from worries and absorb your Self in a productive creation.	
Do one thing, one activity, on action for your Self today. Continue this process each day.	
Forgive your enemies, including enemy number one - your Self. Become your own best friend.	

Problem *Physical Disorder*	**Cause** *Mental Attitude Disorder*
Scleroderma	Defensiveness towards others and in the expression. This produces a resistance mentally, emotionally, and physically where there is a type of armor or shield produced by the body.
Scoliosis	Hiding the true or real identity. Weakness in the identity. Forcing one's Self to be what is desired without having taken the mental and physical action to produce this, without having practiced.
Scratches	Scattering of attention.
Seasickness *see: Motion Sickness*	
Seizures	Attempt to separate Self from emotional overload from others and emotional conditions around the Self. Denial of events that are occurring within the life. Intentional withdrawing of attention from the physical experiences. This causes there to be a misfiring in the brain when there is the withdrawal or tuning out of attention from stimuli being received.
Selfishness	Narrowness of vision. Perpetuating and misusing the stage of infancy.
Senility *see: Alzheimer's Disease*	Refusing to image a future for Self.
Sensory System	Denial of the experiences of the Self.

Remedy *Suggestions for Improvement*	*Personal Notes* *& Observations*
What are you afraid of? Identify your fears. Bring them out into the light of day where you can examine them for what they are, falsehoods.	
Practice one day writing down every thought you have. At the end of the day examine critically every thought. You will begin to know your Self and be aware of what you want to change.	
Concentrate on a blade of grass for ten minutes each day. Concentrate on what others are saying to you in conversation each day.	
The power in correctly identifying events and circumstances in the life is apparent when one beings to change the life for the better due to increased awareness.	
Expand your vision to include others, seeing the influence you have upon others.	
Everyday, create a mental image of a personal desire. Be in the desire. Experience with all five senses until it is real.	
Give your Self credit when credit is due. Appreciate each situation as a real opportunity to progress.	

Problem *Physical Disorder*	**Cause** *Mental Attitude Disorder*
sense of smell	Difficulty with how the attention is used.
sense of taste	same
sense of touch	Turning the attention away from the learning.
sense of sight *see: Eyes*	
sense of hearing *see: Ears*	
Shin(s)	Forcing action.
Shingles	Fighting change. Hesitation in the expression of Self. Defensiveness concerning responding to desires. Need to receive new information from environment instead of blocking it.
Shoulders *see: Joints, Round Shoulders*	
Sickle Cell Anemia	Feeling victimized. Identifying with weakness and blame. Blaming the environment for unfulfilled desires.
Sinus Problems	Self pity. Emotional irresponsibility.
Sinusitis	Self pity. When chronic, Self pity occurs continually because the issue is never resolved.

Remedy *Suggestions for Improvement*	*Personal Notes* *& Observations*
Practice describing one odor each day.	
Practice describing one taste each day.	
Love each experience you create until you find more purpose for living.	
Don't wait until you have to do things. Do them early while you have the control.	
Today do all the activities you have been putting off for the last week. Next week complete all the activities you have been procrastinating on for the past month.	
You are just as good and worthy as anyone. However, only you can prove this to your Self. No one can give it to you.	
Care about your Self enough to honestly share with another exactly how you feel every day.	
Stop feeling sorry for your Self and do something new that is productive. Observe your environment. You will find successes that others have that will stimulate you to create. Don't wait to start. As soon as a desire is realized, act on it.	

Problem *Physical Disorder*	**Cause** *Mental Attitude Disorder*
Skeleton/Skeletal System *see: Bones*	Thinking Self is incapable of using structure to cause motion and mobility.
Skin *see: Hives, Psoriasis, Rash*	Hesitation or insecurity in the expression of the Self.
skin eruptions	Need to appreciate personality and outward expression, not being concerned if others do not. Worry.
Sleeping Disorder *see: Insomnia, Narcolepsy*	Need to release problems of life.
Sleeplessness	Unresolved experiences or unresolved communications.
Slipped Disc	Thinking of Self as too old, weak, or incapable of causing change.
Slowing Down of Bodily Processes	No longer a use for the physical vehicle.
Sluggishness	Defensiveness. No purpose.
Smoking	Need to create comfort with Self when around people and all times. Avoiding the experience of the emotions.
Snoring	Fear of losing control. Hesitation. Mostly physical causes.

Remedy *Suggestions for Improvement*	*Personal Notes* *& Observations*
Consider the structures you are using at the present time, your job or business, your marriage or relationship, your physical body, your car, and others. Do these vehicles or structures aid you to fulfill your desires and needs? Do they improve your quality of living? Are you learning and growing?	
Practice communicating your thoughts and ideas with five different people each day. Listen completely to their responses.	
Be yourself with others; you don't have to fake it.	
Remove your attention from tomorrow's troubles before going to sleep. Place your thoughts on pleasant ideas.	
Act on thoughts that are present throughout the day.	
Think you are old and you are. Think you are young and you are. To stay young continually, change, learn, and grow.	
If you desire to live, then create a purpose for living.	
Stop trying to defend your Self and do what you want to do that is productive.	
What are you hiding? Be honest in sharing your thoughts and who you are. You have much of value to offer.	
Accomplish everything you can today. At night, release the troubles of the day so you will be refreshed and ready for tomorrow.	

Problem *Physical Disorder*	**Cause** *Mental Attitude Disorder*
Solar Plexus	Imbalance between the inner workings and outer workings in the thinking processes, creating emotional vulnerability and difficulty with emotions, particularly reacting when there is a need for response.
Sore Throat see: *Throat, Tonsils*	Indecision or hesitation to act.
Sores	Resistance.
Spasms (muscular) see: *Muscular System*	Scattering of attention.
Spastic Colitis see: *Colon, Colitis, Intestines, Mucous Colon*	Resentment of one's past.
Spinal Curvature see: *Scoliosis, Round Shoulders, Spinal Misalignments*	
Spinal Meningitis	Refusing to admit where one's identity is.
Spine see: *Special Section*	
Spleen	Feeling powerless or all powerful. Fear of loss of anything or anyone that Self is attached to. Difficulty with understanding the quality of power.
Sprains	Scattered attention.

Remedy *Suggestions for Improvement*	*Personal Notes* *& Observations*
Cause undivided attention in order to have clear perception. Then follow with an appropriate response. Create a clear mental image of what is desired to be expressed. Your inner desires are important and need to be shared with others.	
Make determination a part of your life. Don't take no for an answer. Do it now.	
Instead of fighting against, find a cause worth fighting for.	
Give your body and muscles direct commands.	
Forgive your Self by giving to others and aiding others in the present. Learn to love your Self by loving others.	
The identity is within. You are not a physical body. The body is a vehicle for the Real Self. Look into someone else's eyes for five minutes and describe what you discover.	
Image a desire, make a decision and act on it.	
Practice concentrating on a flower ten minutes per day for one month.	

Problem *Physical Disorder*	**Cause** *Mental Attitude Disorder*
Sterility	Refusing to give or receive. Denial concerning one's creative power.
Stiff Neck *see: Muscular System, Neck Problems*	Idea that responsibility is a burden. Trying to be responsible for others. Trying to interfere with other's decisions.
Stiffness	Restriction within the thinking based on holding on to ideas.
Stomach *see: Gastritis, Heartburn, Peptic Ulcer, Ulcers*	Difficulty in receiving new information. Anxiety or worry. When anxiety or worry are present there is not the direction of energy toward a productive end.
Stroke	Refusal to face experiences and conditions within the life. Avoiding conditions, circumstances, or learning in the life. This causes there to be a shutting off of the incoming messages from the brain. The stroke in turn then causes the experience of using and processing the information that has already been received.
Stuttering	Insecurity in communicating thoughts. Doubt in the ability to communicate.
Suicide	Refusal to learn and to cause change.
Swelling *see: Edema, Holding Fluids*	Holding on to ideas that are unproductive.

Remedy *Suggestions for Improvement*	*Personal Notes & Observations*
Discover ways to make this world a better place to live. Invent new ways to use old things. Combine objects in useful ways that will give one a sense of value and productivity.	
Responsibility is the ability to respond to one's inner desires. Identify these.	
How does one create an open mind? Be willing to receive.	
Mentally picture what you desire to occur—not what you fear or don't want to occur.	
Examine your life, what has been fulfilling and productive. What have you always desired to do but have never done? Do it. Practice being who you really want to be.	
Security comes from repeated success and success begins with having a clear mental picture of that which is desired to occur.	
Continual change makes life fun and interesting. Non-growth leads to depression and low desire for life.	
Figure out your benefit for holding on to old ideas that don't work. Then replace them with something better.	

Problem *Physical Disorder*	**Cause** *Mental Attitude Disorder*
Syphilis see: *Venereal Disease*	Resentment of the sexual expression.
Tapeworm	Thinking there can never be enough, that what is present is never enough.
Teeth	Neglect.
Testicles	Difficulty with the masculine expression. Resentment at the idea of having to take care of others. Misuse or misunderstanding of the aggressive expression.
Tetanus see: *Lockjaw*	Being afraid of being controlled by events.
Thalamus see: *Brain*	Confusion in thinking. Need to give undivided attention to receiving impressions from the experiences.
Throat see: *Sore Throat*	Misuse of the understanding of the use of will.
strep throat	Manipulating with the emotions as a misuse of will.
Thrush see: *Yeast Infections*	Irresponsibility in the use of the influence one has with others. Hesitancy in expressing the thoughts.
Thymus	Refusing to mature or difficulty in understanding the process of maturing. Problems with responding to and using adolescence.

Remedy *Suggestions for Improvement*	*Personal Notes & Observations*
Learn mental communication.	
Replace the fear of not having enough with the desire to create more.	
Respect your body as you would take care of any vehicle that served you well.	
Aggressiveness is initiating activity on desires. You chose your body at the beginning of this lifetime. Appreciate that choice.	
Choose what you want to do that will benefit your Self and others and do it. You will then have control of events.	
Taste food. Indentify the ingredients by taste and smell. Describe with words an object seen. Repeat a song.	
Make ten decisions each day different from the previous day and act on them immediately.	
Stop trying to get others to fulfill your desires and start action on your Self on your desires. Then others may want to share in your fulfillment.	
Speak what is on your mind and be willing to listen to others.	
Watch the stages of growth in people. Infancy, adolescence, adulthood and old age/wisdom. Notice the separate qualities of each. Each has value. You cannot stay in any one of these forever. Enjoy where you are, as you are preparing for the next stage.	

Problem *Physical Disorder*	**Cause** *Mental Attitude Disorder*
Thyroid *see: Goiter, Hyperthyroidism, Hypothyroidism*	Misuse of will.
Tics/Twitches *see: Muscular System, Skeletal System*	
Tinnitus	Refusal to hear the thoughts of Self.
Tongue *see: Digestive System*	
Tonsillitis *see: Sore Throat*	Passivity in the use of the will. Anger, because you haven't been decisive enough to fulfill desires.
Toxins	Holding on to unproductive thoughts.
Tuberculosis	Emotional repression from holding on to limited attitudes learned as a child. Identifying with weakness. This attitude interferes with the desire for life and for breath.
Tumors	
malignant	Hatred.
benign	Unproductive, concentrated thoughts.
Ulcers *see: Heartburn, Peptic Ulcer, Stomach Problems*	Worry or anxiety.

Remedy *Suggestions for Improvement*	*Personal Notes* *& Observations*
Picture a goal - move toward your goal with action and determination. Be purposeful about this. Continue with step after step. This is correct use of will.	
Practice concentration and meditation.	
If you do nothing about your desires, you have no one to blame but your Self. So stop being angry at your Self and others and initiate the activity you have been procrastinating on.	
Stop poisoning your Self with your thought. Intentionally think ten productive thoughts each day, verbalizing and recording them.	
What is it that you really want to do with your life? Be honest. Attempt to fulfill your real desire.	
Give to and love others so you learn to love your Self.	
Identify the thoughts and change them to more productive ones.	
Keep your attention in the present.	

Problem *Physical Disorder*	**Cause** *Mental Attitude Disorder*
Unworthiness	Misuse of memory.
Urethritis	Guilt.
Urinary Infections	Guilt.
Urinary System	Regret or guilt.
Uterus	Misunderstanding of the receptive quality in creating.
Vaginitis *see: Female Problems, Leukorrhea*	Insecurity in the feminine expression.
Varicose Veins	Lack of forward motion in the Self and the life. Thinking there is too much to handle. Difficulty with responding to conditions.
Vascular System	Misunderstanding of responsibility.
Vasovagal Attack	Thoughts held for a long period of time that explode in anger.
Veins	Need to be willing to receive stimulus. An evaluation process of the ability of Self to respond, particularly concerning the receptive quality.

Remedy *Suggestions for Improvement*	*Personal Notes & Observations*
Use memory to draw upon productive experiences. Use the memory to separate the past from the present.	
Keep your attention in the present, not the past.	
same as above	
Create opportunities in the present so you can prove to your Self that life is continuous and you have more opportunities.	
Receptivity is expectant non-action. Practice meditation which is the expectant non-action of listening for the answers to the questions given to your subconscious mind.	
Talk to people secure in their own expression. Practice receiving. Learn the power of listening.	
Practice will power and determination. Accept a challenge given by the Self and achieve it.	
Responsibility is freedom. The freedom to respond. The freedom to create.	
Have enough courage to share your thoughts with others long before the pressure builds up.	
Practice graciously reciving compliments and gifts from others. Direct your full attention to receiving impressions through the senses. Learn to be receptive to opportunities in your environment.	

Problem *Physical Disorder*	**Cause** *Mental Attitude Disorder*
Venereal Disease *see: AIDS, Gonorrhea, Herpes, Syphilis*	Disgust or bitterness concerning the sexual expression. Resentment of the responsibility of intimacy.
Vertigo *see: Dizziness*	Refusal to face the conditions around the Self.
Viral Infections *see: Infection*	Indecision.
Vomiting	Refusing to assimilate the experiences of the life.
Vulva	Misunderstanding of the power of receptivity.
Warts	Hesitation in one's learning and growth. Need to give attention to something that is being ignored. Oversensitivity to the environment.
Weakness	Refusal to understand Self worth.
Whiteheads *see: Pimples*	Holding on to unproductive ideas affecting the expression and outer presentation of self.
Whooping Cough	Fear of losing freedom.
Wisdom Tooth impacted	Thinking of the period of childhood as being pleasant and the present conditions and future conditions as being unpleasant.

Remedy *Suggestions for Improvement*	*Personal Notes* *& Observations*
Learn to know your own inner Self and you will not fear being close to others. Rather you will appreciate the opportunity to know a friend.	
Create mental conditions of what you want to occur in your life. Stop living in fear and instead love life.	
Each day, make ten decisions to do something differently from yesterday or last week or the previous month.	
Make learning your number one love.	
Receive the fulfillment of your actions and desires. Be willing to receive.	
Do five activities each day for six months that you have put off doing.	
Practice exercise of gazing at Self in mirror ten minutes each day.	
Unproductive ideas do not give security so replace them with new ideas. Be willing to learn like a child.	
There is a restriction in thinking caused by the believe that freedom means irresponsibility. Believing that one cannot escape situations. Practice responding to conditions rather than running from them.	
The only reason the present is unpleasant is you are not doing what you really want to do.	

Problem *Physical Disorder*	**Cause** *Mental Attitude Disorder*
Wounds *see: Cuts, Injuries*	Holding grudges or resentments in the present experiences.
Wrist *see: Arm, Hand*	Forcing rather than creating purposes for learning. No purpose seen in the activity.
Yeast Infections *see: Thrush*	Insecurity in the feminine expression.

Remedy *Suggestions for Improvement*	*Personal Notes* *& Observations*
The grudge you really hold is against your Self. Forgive your Self for being less than perfect. Perfect means there is no new learning. So no one really wants to be perfect. It would be very boring.	
Purpose is the benefit or learning gained from an experience.	
Nurture your Self and aid others to grow. Give them warmth, concern, caring, and love.	

SPECIAL SECTION

The Spinal Column

The Spinal Column

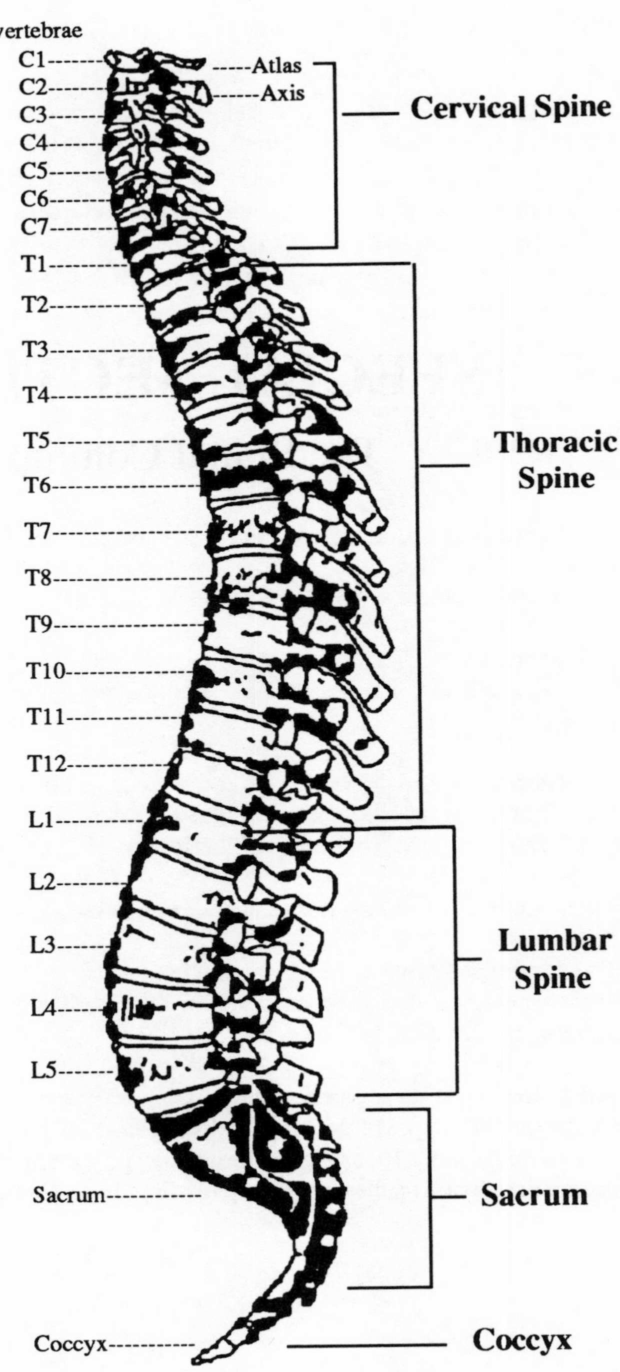

The Spinal Column

In many ways the spinal column and vertebrae mirror the entire system of the human body on a smaller or different type of scale. While reading the disorder-attitudes of the individual vertebra, notice that many attitudes have similiar effects in other parts of the body. For instance, a common attitude affects both a specific vertebra and a specific organ, gland, or system of the body. This is due in part to the activity of the parasympathetic and sympathetic nervous systems which join in nerve trunks along the spine. Spinal fluid moving from the brain to the tailbone also has a role in this physical manifestation of attitudes. This column moves from the tailbone located at the base of the spine to the base of the brain. Overall, difficulties in the spine indicate the need to develop more flexibility within one's Self and the life.

The **Cervical** vertebrae are concerned with and affected by the idea, thought, or will. The original idea. The creation of thoughts and desires, and responsibility for them.

The **Thoracic** vertebrae are closely connected with and influenced by purpose. Causing a direction of thoughts and desires that is a fulfillment of the ideals of Self.

The **Lumbar** vertebrae work with the activity in bringing the thought into manifestation or mobility. The Lumbar is associated with causing action to fulfill the desires that produce the understanding of power and forward motion.

The **Coccyx** is a manifestation of either extreme passivity or extreme forcing.

The **Sacrum** is similar to the Coccyx but less extreme. This arises because one waits for external factors to move Self in one direction or another rather than initating action in the Self.

The following pages list each spinal vertebra separately. With each listing is a notation of the types of thinking producing susceptibility to misalignment or injury. Suggestions for changing the quality and patterns of thinking for each disorder are found on the right hand page directly across from these notations.

CERVICAL	**Ideal.** The action of thinking. The forming of thought concerning action that is desired to be taken. Misunderstanding of responsibility regarding how to use the will to respond and the idea that responsibility is a burden. This would also relate to thoughts, ideas, and will. Intelligence, or the ability to receive information, to send information, to process it and to create with it. Sense of identity and responding to abilities with the will or will power.
C-1	Restriction of the thinking processes. This causes one to think he is being pressured by conditions and circumstances.
C-2	Difficulty in perception. Limitation of imagination due to incomplete or vague thoughts.
C-3	Restriction in receiving information. Insecurity.
C-4	Restriction in receiving information. Misuse of memory. Self pity. Comparing present thoughts with memories of disappointment or failure or other experiences that inhibit fulfillment of desires.
C-5	Restriction in receiving information. Need to communicate. Speak your thoughts so you are willing to receive the words and thoughts of others. Insecurity as to the identity of Self in relationship to others.
C-6	Restriction in thinking. Specifically, unwillingness to complete a thought in regards to giving the full attention to a mental creation. Being overwhelmed by too many thoughts without a direction. Need to exercise the will in order to think and pursue one thought at a time.
C-7	Need to use will to set desires into motion. Thinking the Self to be weak, due to passivity in setting desires into motion.

Change every negative or unproductive thought to a productive thought. Write a list of your ten most wanted desires. Make this list in order starting with number one as your strongest desire working toward number ten as your tenth strongest desire. Read this daily.

Examine your thoughts. Get out of your rut. Stop being habitual and do something different. Change every negative or unproductive thought to a productive thought.

Go to lectures and hear people speak on subjects you are not informed or knowledgeable in.

Go to listen to ten speakers lecture that have an opposing or differing view from your own. Find at least ten percent of the lecture you can agree with.

Try and experiment with new thoughts and ideas. Listen to and learn new ideas each day.

Share your ideas, concepts and thoughts with others. You may be a great inventor.

Choose a thought and completely describe it with words that another can completely understand.

Visualize your desires completely and in detail. Share them with others. Initiate some type of action toward fulfillment of these desires each day.

THORACIC	**Purpose.** Purposefulness or intention of thought in terms of its creation and manifestation, particularly manifestation. Anxiety concerning the ability of the Self to fulfill the desires of Self.
T-1	Relative to the beginning of initiating purpose. Worry about the ability of Self to overcome limitations or obstacles. Physical activity without mental direction. Refusal to use the imagination to visualize how to use challenges.
T-2	Purpose in regards to identity. Responsibility for learning. Difficulty in using will power to be responsible for the desires of Self. Worry concerning the future.
T-3	Purpose in regards to Self expression. Worry or anxiety concerning performing adequately or living up to the ideals of Self, or ability of Self to cause forward motion. Fear of failure. Trying to fulfill the desires of others rather than Self.
T-4	Difficulty in purposefulness as it relates to understanding. Direct the thought into creating in the environment rather than trying to control people. Making a burden of responsibility rather than using responsibility to create freedom. Need to understand that responsibility is an expression of Self that provides for a greater expansion of Self.
T-5	Purpose or intention in regards to responsibility. Purpose for living. You are responsible for causing learning to occur. Anxiety concerning the ability of Self to cause forward motion.
T-6	Difficulty in assimilating experiences. Fear of rejection. Attention is directed toward how Self will be perceived by others and this produces a turning away from determining the learning Self will receive from an experience.
T-7	Purpose or intention in regards to understanding the learning in an experience. Holding onto ideas of the past restricting giving thus limiting one's ability to receive from others.

Form a productive purpose for every thought you have. Become flexible in your thinking and actions. When with others, cooperate.

Ask yourself each day, "What is the purpose for my activity and my day?" Create an answer.

Ask your Self, "What benefit will I derive from each desire I undertake?" Answer this question.

Create desire based upon what *you* *want to happen in* *your* *life. Communicate your desires to others for the express purpose of allowing them to aid you in fulfilling your desires.*

There is a need to change, learn and grow from the fulfillment of your desires so you become a better person.

Ask your Self, "What is my life's purpose?" Set yearly and lifetime goals. Have a purpose of growth in these goals.

Ask your Self ten times each day in ten different experiences, "What did I learn from that experience?" Keep a journal of your discoveries.

Learn from your mistakes and successes. Create a better you in everything you do.

T-8	Purpose in regards to an inflow and outflow, whether it manifests as communication or energy. Difficulty in giving and receiving. Responsibility of assimilation of learning in experiences. Trying to please others. When the mind is directed toward pleasing others there is interference in putting into practice what is desired to be learned.
T-9	Need to achieve a balance in giving and receiving. Responsibility to use the situation that is present. Holding onto guilts or condemnations.
T-10	Responsibility to release the past so giving and receiving and learning can occur. Purposefulness in relation to external factors in regard to what is understood and completely learned from the experiences. Thinking there is something owed to Self rather than understanding how to pay the debts the Self owes. Holding onto blame of others rather than identifying Self as cause.
T-11	Need to establish what one's intention is in terms of learning. Fear of the unknown due to living in past hurts.
T-12	Responsibility for discrimination in terms of reasoning and understanding Self as cause. One's thoughts begin the cause of one's life. Blaming others when you need to look at Self as cause. Need to discriminate what are the thoughts of Self and what are the thoughts of others.

Learn to give. People have difficulty receiving because they refuse to give. Purposely and intentionally give three times each day for one month. Your reward will come from the universe.

Whenever someone offers to help you, learn to receive and accept their offer of friendship.

Living in the past produces no-thing. The present is where you create a purpose for living and purpose for a lifetime. Every time your thought goes to an unpleasant or negative situation from the past, say out loud three times, "My thoughts are in the present and I can create my desires in the present."

Every time a fear occurs in your mind, say out loud three times, "I am on a voyage of discovery. I am making exciting, new, and important discoveries."

Sit down and honestly evaluate your thoughts and attitudes determining which are constructive and which are not. Your thought of today is your life of tomorrow. Examine each goal you hold to insure there is a constructive purpose for your goal that will benefit you and many others.

LUMBAR **Activity.** Necessary actions to be taken. Part of this is in regards to responding to manifested desires, part of it is in regards to initiating new creations. Misunderstanding power. There is action in the conscious mind of forming a desire, drawing upon memory of experiences or information that is interpreted as being in conflict with the desire and seeing or believing that these conflicting images will inhibit the fulfillment of the original desire. Need for creative forward motion. Need to use the ability of Self for full expression, motion, movement, and manifestation of the thoughts and ways of thinking of the Self in order to use and apply the creativity of the Self. When one holds onto the past or is reacting to others desires this creates in the Self an overall sense of powerlessness with conditions and circumstances.

L-1 Thoughts and actions don't match. Difficulty in cooperating with the desires of Self in terms of the actions of Self being different from intentions. Thinking that Self is powerless.

L-2 Refusal to use the ability to cause forward movement. Restriction in expressing influence. Attachment to something that is no longer needed. Thinking the environment controls Self rather than causing motion to produce what is desired in the environment. Feeling powerless regarding the environment.

L-3 Conflict issue concerning attachment to the past. An object or situation from the past is still desired but this no longer serves a purpose for forward motion, learning, and growth in the life. Feeling powerless in relationships with others.

L-4 Difficulty, attachment, or holding back on the ability to create action that is compatible with what has already been set into motion. Restriction regarding acting on desires. Need to have a willingness to respond to conditions as they exist. Sense of powerlessness due to blaming others for current situation. Need to choose how to respond with action rather than making others the causal factor for existing conditions.

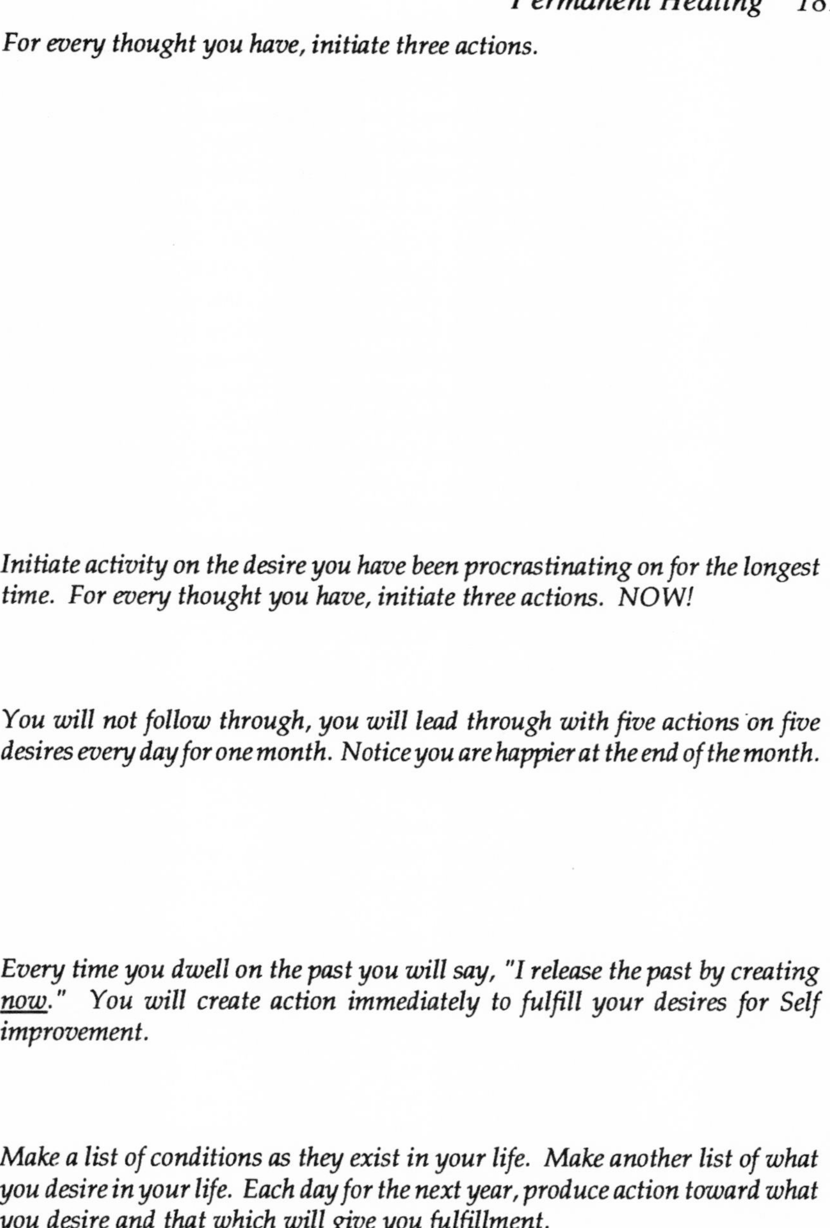

For every thought you have, initiate three actions.

Initiate activity on the desire you have been procrastinating on for the longest time. For every thought you have, initiate three actions. NOW!

You will not follow through, you will lead through with five actions on five desires every day for one month. Notice you are happier at the end of the month.

Every time you dwell on the past you will say, "I release the past by creating now." You will create action immediately to fulfill your desires for Self improvement.

Make a list of conditions as they exist in your life. Make another list of what you desire in your life. Each day for the next year, produce action toward what you desire and that which will give you fulfillment.

L-5 Need to be able to respond to what is occurring within the Self and within the life with action and forward motion. Conflicting ideas of Self from the past and present both held within the mind. This creates a difficulty in causing any type of forward motion.

COCCYX Thinking there is not the capability within the Self to create what is desired. The responsibility in terms of the coccyx is to cause motion consistently in order to prove to Self the strength of Self.

SACRUM Thinking of Self as physical only. The responsibility here is to understand and pursue the awareness of the creativity of the Self by using thought.

Whatever needs doing, do it now. Be in the now, cause action now. The present is the only time you can change or grow. Be in the eternal present.

Practice an activity that requires endurance more than strength.

Meditate each day on your next step in life. "Where do I go from here?" is the question you ask, and listen for the answer in meditation. Once you receive an answer, pursue it vigorously.

Cranial or Skull Plates and Sutures

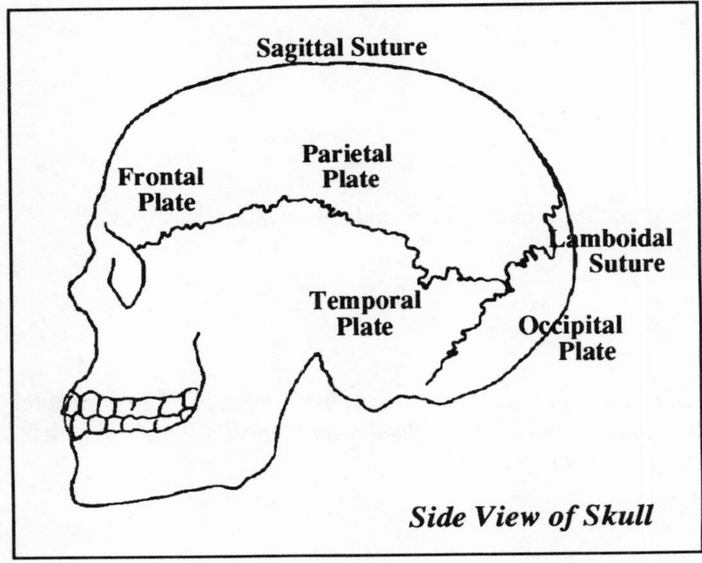

Side View of Skull

Cranium Misalignment of cranial plates is created by pressure experienced in the action of thinking.

Frontal Misalignment occurs in this area when attention is scattered producing failure in the use of the imagination. When the attention is diverted toward what one does not want to occur in the future worry is experienced. Without the use of proper perspective, there is no order to the thoughts thus producing the idea or image of being overwhelmed. This causes pressure. Refusal to exercise the imagination fosters insecurity concerning the capability to reason and express Self fluently.

Temporal This area of the skull relates to higher perception and the manner in which concepts are perceived. Misalignment occurs when perception and receptivity are restricted. This creates an ignorance of the purpose in this lifetime. You are denying your inner authority and feeling pressured by the people in positions of authority. You ignore the awareness the Self does hold and strain to find that awareness outside of the Self.

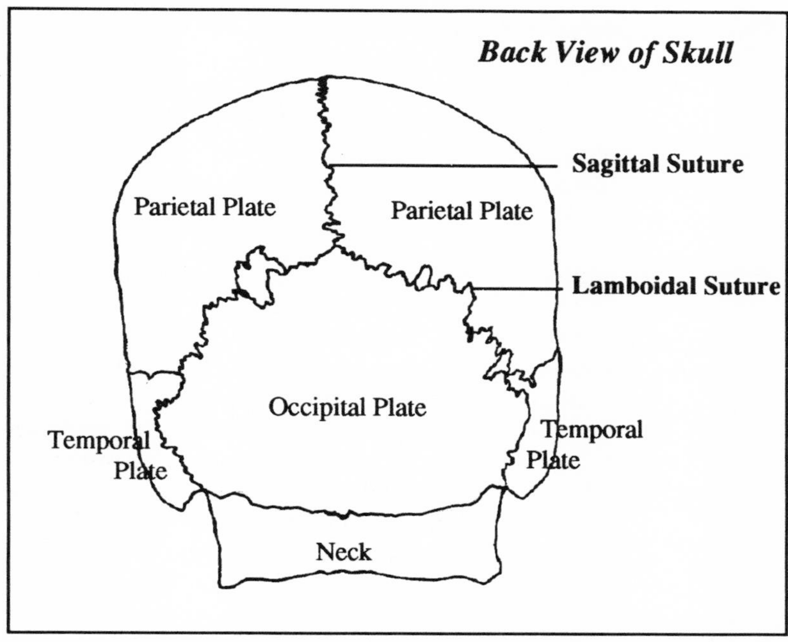

When this occurs, you need to give attention to understanding reasoning and the spiritual nature of Self.

Practice listening. When listening to another do not think and don't formulate your response while listening to another. Rather, give your whole attention to receiving what the other person has to say. Then practice saying it back, out loud, word for word.

Meditate for twenty minutes each day. Practice meditation as expectant listening to your inner, higher Self. Write in a journal what you receive in meditation. Apply it in your life for your betterment and the betterment of others.

Occipital Misuse of memory concerning what has been made a permanent part of Self. There are reactions to images stored from the past. This creates impediments to using memory in the present time period. Reaction to old memory patterns inhibits you from creating the future.

Parietal Difficulties in thinking and the cognitive or reasoning ability, particularly in regards to communication. Your inner and outer life are disconnected. You feel external conditions are limiting your freedom because you hesitate in decision making. This creates a feeling of being pressured by external conditions and defensiveness in the thought processes. Fantasizing rather than using the imagination interferes with your use of memory and information organization. Difficulty with touching others and the environment.

Sagittal When you are unable to communicate your mental images accurately, misalignment will occur in this area. Coordination of mental images and verbal description is a key element for this area of the skull. An imbalance between the physical experiences and the accurate verbalization of them exists. Gathering tremendous quantities of information in the brain without the willingness to apply this information in the life will create misalignment in this area.

Lamboidal When you refuse to speak your thoughts you create impediments to improving your thinking processes. This causes misalignment in this area. Difficulty describing in words what has been experienced through the senses reduces your ability to communicate clearly. You are reacting to what is received by the senses rather than using your attention to separate and identify the information.

Practice concentration ten minutes a day on the object of your choice such as the tip of your finger.
Try new activities and hobbies to discover your hidden talents and abilities.

Communication is one of the qualities that separates mankind from the animals. Therefore, create a place or find a topic or subject you can teach and do so. Teach others and also lecture. This will place you in a position of communicating with many more people and to a greater degree.

Join a group, club, or organization and become an active member. Learn to work with people to accomplish projects that would be difficult for one person to accomplish alone. Learn the power of people working together.

Each day for one month choose ten different physical places that you visit or travel to or are in and observe them. Then spend five minutes describing each place or environment using all five senses to describe what it looks, smells like, sounds like, tastes like, and feels like. This is learning to communicate the whole picture.

PERMANENT HEALING
Section III

Quantum Mechanics of Healing

Many times in my career, I have witnessed individuals displaying specific attitudes in their manner of expression: verbally, mentally, emotionally, and physically. I would also watch these people develop illnesses to match their attitudes. As an educator, I have taught thousands of people what attitudes create disorders in their physical bodies. Sometimes they would change, grow, and expand their limited thinking and following this, experience permanent healing. Others maintained their habits and limited, unproductive ways of thinking and invariably would create illness in the body.

The mind-body connection is sufficiently established in the public's mind to such a degree that more and more people desire to receive and use the information presented here. Some of the attitudes and their physical illness connection listed in Section II may be quite apparent to you at first reading while others may require some reasoning, contemplation, and examination.

Once you have practiced and trained yourself in the skill of recognizing an attitude associated with an illness, the wisdom contained within these pages will be at your fingertips. Your eyes will be opened and you will view life in new, more expansive ways. You will no longer see yourself as a victim of life. Rather, you will recognize that you are the controller and director of your life. What you make of your life, pleasant or unpleasant, depends on you. Your health depends on you. Ultimately, our susceptibility to illness and disease depends on our attitudes. Negative, destructive, and unproductive thoughts create a susceptibility in the body for destruction and organizational breakdown. This breakdown we call dis-ease or illness.

People tend to confuse in their thinking the issue of blame and responsibility. The idea of having created their disease seems abhorrent to them. They think it means they must be a terrible person to have done this. If you already have a low sense of self worth, the last thing you want to do is to admit your guilt in creating illness in the body. Fortunately, there is another more productive method of viewing the situation. Instead of blame, "I did something terrible," we can consider illness from the point of desiring to understand cause and respond accordingly. Responsibility is the ability to respond to your inner, most heartfelt desires to learn, grow and improve your life, including your physical body.

As you use this book, learn to have compassion for your Self. Recognize it requires effort to improve and to change old, outworn attitudes. To forgive others, or your Self, is to release them, or yourself, from the past. You cannot change the past but you can adjust your current response to it. Remember, in order for a disease to find a home, you must provide a place for it with your mind. Knowing this, you can eradicate any unproductive attitude and replace it with the changed, more expansive you.

The boundaries of your mind are not limited to the borders of your body. It is important to know not only that you have created your present condition, but also to know how you have created that condition. For only by knowing how to change can we improve, adjust, and develop the new, more improved Self.

Fears and doubts are two of the greatest limitations. However, when you allow the self-imposed, supposedly protective, walls to come down then your world expands causing remote opportunities and possibilities to become probabilities. Two people can go through the same experience and interpret it completely differently. One person may react with anger and resentment while the other responds with joy and happiness. The choice is yours because we each create our own view of reality.

We are constantly bombarded with a myriad of sense impressions from our environment as well as a vast array of desires and thoughts. The manner in which you interpret these impulses becomes your individual reality. Each person puts his own interpretation on the data that comes in through the senses. We listen to the world selectively. It is our duty to still the mind and focus the attention in order to gain the most from each experience and learn to expand our awareness of reality and Self.

The dishonest conscious ego will see the world as a dangerous place and something to fear. The world will be one of duality between "I" and "them". An honest conscious ego and a focused mind perceive the Self as part of nature and the universe. There is a feeling of oneness with life. Many have experienced this feeling of oneness during meditation. It is our duty to develop this experience of connectedness into a permanent realization of the importance of the influence each of us have on everyone else. The great value of a beneficial influence is seen when we examine the greatest recovery factor for people who have experienced heart attacks.

The most significant recovery factor for male heart attack victims in many cases is whether they perceived their wives loved them. Love is a thought, an expression of Self, a caring to which the emotions of warmth and tenderness attach themselves. The desire and willingness to change creates an opening in awareness that makes life a much more expansive place to live.

People do not have to get sick or age as they grow older. Aging, as many people recognize, is a factor of one's attitude. For many years I taught a man in his 70's who was more active and healthy than many people half his age. Al was also more willing to change, adjust, and release old ways of thinking than most people half his age. He practiced the meditation I taught him over one hour each day. In addition, Al practiced concentration, dream interpretation, memory exercises, and reading lessons on Self awareness daily. He was disciplined. He stilled his mind and directed his thought to productive ends.

In teaching students to change and transform themselves, I have seen many progress through initiations and gain the most beautiful experience of watching their world expand beyond their accustomed limits. This is bliss. Bliss is the conscious connection between Self and Mind, between Mind and matter. The consciousness of the Mind can permanently heal the lower form of consciousness of the body. The body and conscious mind at times hold onto what is comfortable, what you have become used to and accustomed to because it has not changed. However, it is forward motion that brings change and happiness. Illness is an indication war is going on inside you, a war between growth and non-change. However, there is no one to fight against but yourself. Why would you want to fight against your Self?

Anytime there is spontaneous remission of cancer there is always an incredible jump forward in one's awareness. If you break your arm, you have it set and put it in a cast. It is the intelligence, the consciousness of the body, that then takes over and causes the bones to mend together. It is consciousness or directing intelligence that causes the arm to mend, and this is also true with cancer.

Physically, cancer is out-of-control cells in the body. It is similar to an out-of-control person who exhibits anti-social behavior by trying to dominate everyone in his environment due to Self insecurities. A cancer cell reproduces itself without check, no longer cooperating with the rest of the body, only listening to its own distorted DNA. The reason this occurs and how it is created is due to the attitude causing cancer which is hate; extreme hate or hate that has been held in the thoughts for a long time. A person who is filled with hate will have either anti-social behavior towards others (such as anger, rage, fear, disgust and antagonism) or in many cases these thoughts will be repressed and held within. In this way it is seen that *specific* attitudes affect the body *specifically* because the body-mind is one unit.

Our attitudes create constant change within our bodies. On a subatomic, atomic, molecular, and cellular level the body is never the same today as it was yesterday. Ninety-eight percent of the atoms in your body were not there one year ago. The skin you create is new every month. You gain a new stomach lining every four days. Doesn't it make sense to produce healthier tissue and a healthy body by directing the production of the replacement tissue with productive attitudes?

You form a new liver every six weeks. A new skeleton is manufactured every three months. Atoms pass regularly back and forth between the cell walls throughout your body instructed by your directing intelligence. The body is ever changing. Movement and change are the standards for the body. Your degree of understanding and use of the attitudes of the mind enable you to change disorder attitudes to those creating order and improvement.

The brain is constantly sending messages or communication in the form of electrical impulses via the nerve trunks of the body and outward to all tissues. It is now known that the central nervous system sends message throughout the body by way of neurons. Moreover, it also sends messages through the immune system.

Neuro-transmitters act in our body as communicators enabling neurons in the brain to communicate with the rest of the body. Neuro-transmitters move from the brain to every organ in our body communicating our happiness or sadness, emotions, memories, perceptions, attitudes and thoughts. These are chemically coded messages.

The mind controls the brain. The brain affects and controls the body. Thus, it is seen that mental attitudes affect and create order or disorder in the physical body. The discovery of neuro-transmitters shows the interaction of mind and body is one of continual change. Because of this, the body has an incredible capability to communicate from cell to cell.

Receptors or receiving stations for inter-body communication have been discovered during the 1980's on cells in the immune system. Receptors reside on white blood cells called monocytes whose function is to receive communication or messages from the brain. So not only does the central nervous system relay messages from brain to body and body to brain, but this communication also occurs in the immune system and other systems of the body! Neuro-peptides, and receptors for them, exist in many organs of the body such as the kidneys, stomach, and intestines creating brain-body connections.

Therefore, when the mental attitude is indecisive, the attitude is relayed through the brain to the body. Since indecision produces no motion, it is as if you laid down to die. This in turn causes a weakening or sluggishness, and lowers the efficiency of the immune system thus paving the way for the cold and flu virus to take root. Self pity acts in a similar manner on the immune system creating sinusitis and reccurring sinus disorders. Cells are intelligent. They have localized intelligence with a kind of instinct to communicate with other cells.

The mind also communicates to the body concerning fat and weight problems. The vast majority of people who go on diets gain all the weight back once they go off the diet. This is because eliminating food or changing the diet is a physical attempt to remedy what is a mental situation. The thought patterns inducing these people to overeat, thus creating sluggishness in moving foods through the digestive and eliminatory systems, have not changed. In order for there to be permanent healing and a permanent cure, the thought pattern or attitudes must be transformed into a higher state of awareness of what is good for the whole Self.

Messenger molecules in the body such as neuro-peptides and neuro-transmitters show how a thought or attitude and an accompanying body reaction can form a cause-effect relationship. The neuropeptide is directed by and motivated by thoughts. This is a crossover from thought to matter, from mind to body. To crossover from matter to mind, from the physical to the mental, we may use terms that describe the world which is smaller than the body, smaller than a cell of the body, smaller than a molecule or an atom and penetrate into the sub-atomic realm of activity.

As we investigate the world of the infinitely small, we discover the changeover point from matter or physical to thought energy. The name given to the branch of physics exploring these subatomic particles is quantum physics or quantum mechanics. Quantum is a word used to describe a quantity of a substance that can no longer be reduced or sized down and still be that same substance. For example, an electron cannot be cut in half to form two halves of an electron. If you break an electron in half, you create different subatomic particles that bear the qualities of free will and thought more than those of physical matter. All forms of energy are based on a quantum unit. That is the smallest constituent part. It cannot be broken down any smaller.

This subatomic level existing at the changeover point between mind and matter, thought and physical, is the site at which healing of a permanent or miraculous kind must occur. It is your consciousness, your attitude, that creates the change at this level which later affects the physical matter of your body.

An atom is composed of three elementary particles. Two of these, the neutron and proton, are housed in the nucleus of the atom. The third particle, the electron, revolves around the nucleus. The electron carries a negative charge. The proton carries a positive charge and the neutron is neutral. Subatomic particles such as electrons, which travel in orbits around the nucleus of an atom, and a nucleus consisting of protons and neutrons which make up the core of an atom, occupy less than one percent of the space of an atom. This means atoms consist of more than 99% empty space. This means our dense physical bodies are actually more than 99% empty space! Our bodies are as void or have as much empty space proportionately as intergalactic space. Since our bodies are mostly empty space, the dynamic energy interplays throughout the atom are guided by the consciousness of attitudes that act upon those atoms and molecules.

In order to explain further how thought transforms and acts on matter, use this Mind Chart diagram of the divisions of mind, the dimensions of consciousness.

Mind Chart

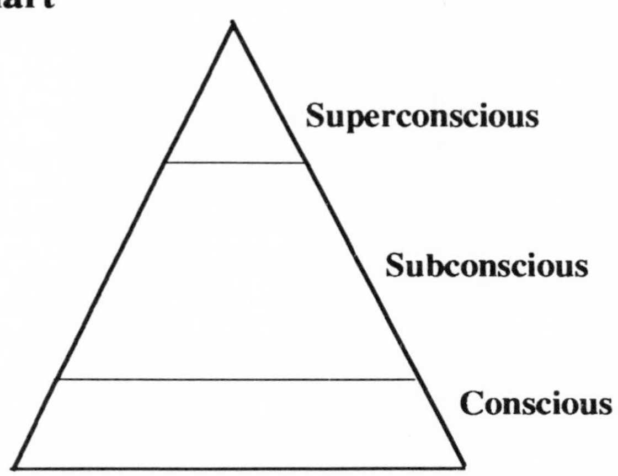

The thoughts and attitudes created in your conscious mind affect your inner Self, the subconscious mind. In the subconscious mind, they combine, gathering substance until they become concentrated enough to "pop" back into existence at the sub-atomic level. The idea of particles popping into and out of existence has been recognized in modern physics for over 50 years.

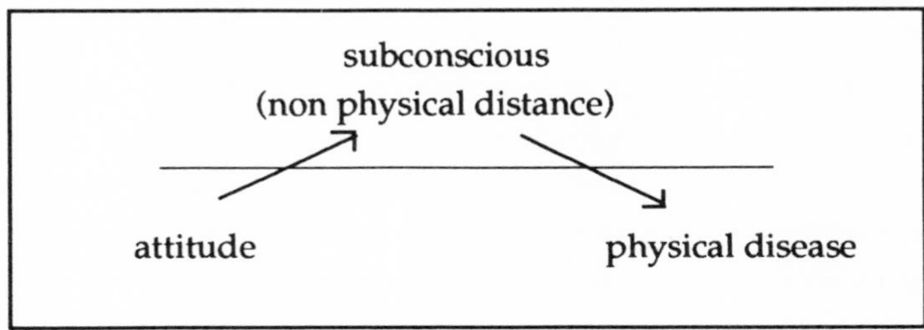

Think a thought, any thought, such as "white house", and a large number of brain cells have to fire. This is enough in itself to have a profound affect on the rest of the body.

The quantum theory of the nature of light developed by Einstein, Planck, Bohr, Heisenberg, and other great physicists in the early part of this century showed how matter could change to mind substance, time into space, and mass into energy and convert back again. At the subatomic level, matter and energy proceed from non-energy and non-matter, which I call thought affected by individuality and free will.

Subatomic particles defy the idea of physical causality. For example, when two subatomic particles have spins matched to one another, you can move them thousands or even millions of light years apart and they will still respond immediately to a change in the spin of the other "twin" particle. This indicates faster than the speed of light effects. This is termed non-local causality because it is faster than physical laws or the laws of physics permit. However, it is in agreement with the universal laws of mind and with Metaphysics which teaches that thought is faster than the speed of light and can be instantaneous, anywhere in the universe. In fact, Bell's theorem in physics accepts the inter-connectedness principle. According to Bell's theorem, everyone and everything in the universe is connected on some level. I call this place or level the inner dimension of mind or subconscious mind.

We live in a universe packed with energy. Because a photon (unit of light) is without mass and travels at the speed of light, it can move out of physical existence into the world of unseen energy (the inner mind) and back into the world of matter. Many of these unseen particles of the universe are called virtual energy, or virtual particles, because they wait in the inner dimensions of mind for the opportunity to be drawn into the physical universe by man's desires and will to create.

Emptiness of matter, fullness of unseen energy, interactions and processes, are the beginning place for everything that exists. We experience and draw upon this inner dimensional power every time we visualize or create thought in our minds. It is this energy that eventually affects the body for health or disease. And it is this ability that can cause permanent healing.

All physical matter seems to cease at the infinitesimal size known as Planck's limit which is 10^{-33} cubic centimeters. Anything smaller than this does not exist physically. In fact, this is the limit of the physical. This is the change-over point from physical to thought. The physical causal relationship between events breaks down at anything smaller than this. A distance in space can be traversed by a particle of matter without being synchronized with a piece of time. Events occur at infinite velocity. They traverse physical space with no time elapsed at this level.

Subconscious
no physically measured time or space

A distance B
physical

The verbal interpretation of quantum theory, the Metaphysics of quantum mechanics, has not been clearly stated in over fifty years since it was first formulated. Physicists present physics. However a teacher of Self and mind, that is metaphysics, practices communicating and teaching the universal truths as a part of their daily routine. They are practiced and accomplished at communicating in day-to-day physical terms in a manner anyone can understand, these timeless truths, laws and principles. It is due to the timelessness of this need on the part of humanity to know these truths and because I have been teaching and practicing Metaphysics for over 15 years that I will now bring the two together in a way that the man on the street can comprehend.

We have heard since the 1960's the statement we are all one. Well, I tell you, we are not all one. We are each unique individuals. However, the oneness or unity occurs in the interconnectedness of all of us one to the other. In other words, what any one person says, does, or thinks affects everyone else. The higher anyone reaches in their soul evolution, the more powerful are the vibrations they emit. As a person meditates and practices concentration exercises his thoughts become more focused and thereby more powerful, affecting the whole of humanity in a more powerful and all inclusive manner. Therefore his perception and awareness of interconnectedness increases.

To understand this universal interconnectedness, it is necessary to present factors concerning the subatomic particle known as the electron. It is not possible to say with certainty exactly where an electron will be within an electron cloud or orbit because the universe is one of infinite possibilities. It is our free will that interacts with and on the universal motion. It is our free will to direct our thoughts that effects this motion causing our reality to mold itself around us. On the subatomic level, the result is instantaneous. On the level of our day to day experiences, the effect of our thoughts often takes longer to be felt in our lives, but this is only due to the fact that there needs to be a build up of subatomic particles in order to generate enough of an energy field moving in a certain direction to cause the matter of our physical existence to change, and affect us in our day to day lives.

According to Heisenberg, one of the great physicists involved in developing modern physics, we can never know with accuracy both the time an event occurs and the energy involved with it. The reason we can never know both the time an event occurs and the energy involved in it with great accuracy is due to the relativity effect. Relativity says that as we move faster, time slows down for the person moving faster. Compare this with Metaphysics which teaches that when any person causes greater and more directed forward motion in their life, they identify more with vertical or mental time rather than horizontal or physical time. Therefore, one who is in motion, constantly producing, learning and growing actually finds all the time they need to produce what they want with their life. This is because as we grow and change, physical, horizontal time slows down. We identify with vertical time which is based on learning and growth, and the speed of thought which is near instantaneous rather than identifying with horizontal, physical time which is limited by the speed of light, 186,000 miles per second.

An object gets shorter in the direction of its motion, until approaching the speed of light, an object's length or distance contracts to a point. As a person's mental motion increases (his ability to create) distance ceases to be a limitation. Time and space come under the control of a thinker, a creator, and there is enough of both to accomplish all of one's desires until in the end one achieves desirelessness as concerns the physical experience. Since space and time are no longer seen as different but are unified in relativistic physics we can see that it is not so important where we travel horizontally (physical space) as where we travel vertically (mental space) from the world of subatomic particles to the outer fringes of the universe.

Our ability to perceive reality using only the five senses is very limited and uses only a small portion of the electro-magnetic light spectrum (less than 5%). To believe that the reality we observe with the senses is the total or even close to the total reality is absurd. Through the experience of teaching mind and Metaphysics for many years, I have found that the habitual limitations people place on themselves are seen to be ridiculous once that person has grown, changed, and developed their intelligence, awareness, and perception beyond their old, worn out, limited concepts.

Geometry and mathematics are devices mankind has created to expand our ability to understand the universe we live in beyond the extent that our five senses alone permit. However, they are abstractions. Quantum mechanics however delves deeper and deeper into the true nature of reality, both the physical and the mental, matter and mind. At the subatomic level, the length of the lifetime of a particle increases with the speed of that particle. Thus a photon, which is a massless particle, is always traveling at the speed of light. Therefore a photon exists forever unless it is annihilated by collision with another particle. The one who has increased his inner motion and raised his consciousness to the point of maximum speed in understanding the nature of Self, creation, and reality-mind lives in eternity. He exists for all intents and purposes in eternity and he experiences life everlasting. This is heaven on earth. However, the lifetime of a particle decreases the slower its motion. This is true for people also. The more we create negative habitual and limited thoughts, the easier it is for dis-ease and illness to come into our body, our body ages quicker and we experience a shorter lifetime just like the subatomic particle.

Light is made of elementary particles known as photons. Pairs of positrons and electrons with a positive and negative charge can be created by photons which are units or packets or quanta of light. Creation of the aggressive and receptive principles of creation occur through the medium of these units of light. In fact, it can be seen that all matter and the whole of the physical universe we experience with the five senses began as light.

The electrons are arranged in clouds, shells, or orbits about the nucleus. The more we compress these particles, the more reaction in terms of motion we observe. This restlessness of matter in reaction to confined space is the same restlessness people experience when they confine themselves to limited ways of thinking. This dissatisfaction with the present state of affairs in one's life stimulates greater activity on the part of a person desiring change and growth to go beyond the limited confines of their life and to seek out a new more expanded consciousness and way of life. In fact, this is exactly what one experiences before entering on the path of enlightenment. The person experiences a dissatisfaction with their life, a lack of fulfillment, and a feeling that they are somehow different from everybody else.

The universe is not static, but expanding. Therefore in order to find fulfillment in an expanding universe, you yourself must cause an expansiveness in your reasoning, intuition, and enlightenment. The more distant a galaxy is from our Milky Way galaxy, the faster it moves away from us. This means the only way you can ever truly know the whole universe is to expand your consciousness at the speed of thought which is greater than the speed of light, to encompass the entire universe. At this point you have achieved compatibility with your creator, the maker of the universe.

Relativity posits an expanding universe that is curved, not flat, and one that is expanding into a higher reality. Metaphysicists call these higher dimensions subconscious mind and superconscious mind.

The full meaning of space-time in relativistic physics is that space and time are fully equivalent. They are unified in a four-dimensional continuum. We live in a four dimensional universe, not a three dimensional universe. Therefore to understand and comprehend the universe we must understand time which is one of the four dimensions of the physical. In order to understand time one must make full use of the time a person has each day. We live in the eternal now. Horizontal time as a sequence of linear events, such as the seasons changing each year or 24 hours in a day, is a construct of the conscious mind and its horizontal thinking.

Real time is vertical and is measured in relation to the advancement of one's thoughts or, in other words, the steps of evolution towards enlightenment and universal or cosmic consciousness (see diagrams).

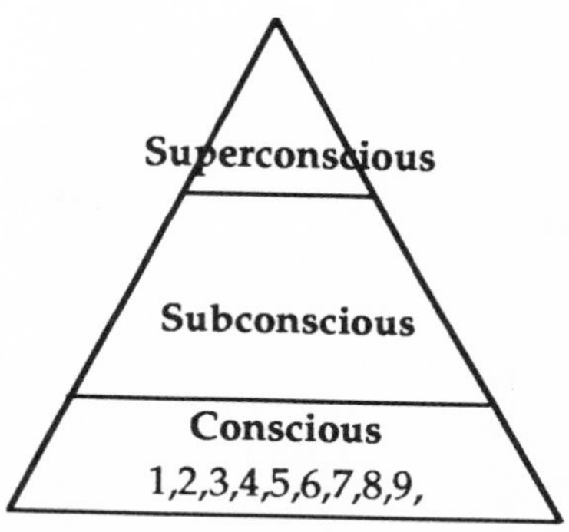

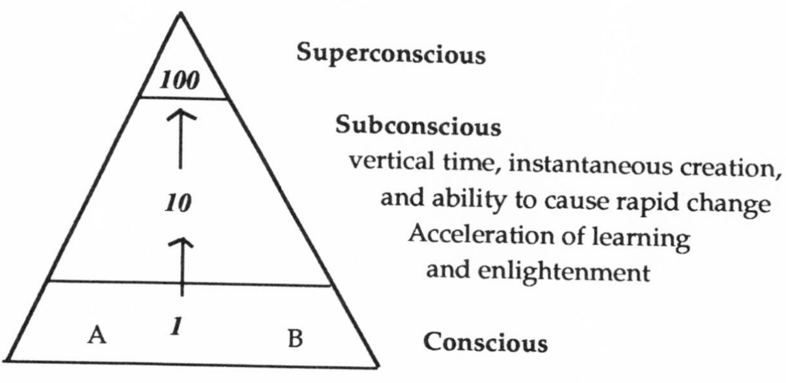

The top diagram illustrates the person who identifies only with the conscious mind, physical, horizontal time as a linear sequence of events. This person has to plod along, go through all steps one through 10 in order to accomplish his goal. This requires lots of physical time. The enlightened person however by-passes or transcends this physical time, identifies with vertical time and accomplishes steps one through 10 by going directly from one to 10. The realization or learning is quickened. This then is the meaning of omnipresence and omniscience. This is the all-knowing, where past, present and future come together. Such a one lives in the eternal now.

Matter is made up of energy. The conservation of energy is one of the fundamental laws of physics. No violation of this law has ever been observed. Therefore, when matter is destroyed or changed it becomes energy and when energy is destroyed or changed it becomes matter. $E=mc^2$. Mass is the measure of the inertia of an object. Inertia equals resistance to being accelerated. The longer a person remains the way they are without learning and growing, the more difficult it is to change and move beyond old habits and previously accepted limitations. The laws of physics concerning inertia have a direct counterpart for the individual called mental inertia.

Relativity theory says that mass is another form of energy. Therefore, when we apply enough energy in the direction of causing growthful improvement and enlightenment in our life, the result will be that we will overcome the inertia of our old limited way of being. Mass (and therefore our lives) is not static but rather is one of motion and change. To create fulfillment in life, we quicken this change and motion in the direction of our inner desires and ideals for Self fulfillment. The discovery that mass is a form of energy aids us in understanding that the nature of the physical is change. We can change with it and even cause greater change. We can build control and fulfillment in life, or we can resist change, be out of control, and find our life filled with sadness and despair.

Atoms consist of particles and these particles are not made of physical, material matter but rather are dynamic energy patterns continually transforming themselves. Your life is meant to be a dynamic process of energy exchange from one level to a higher level. It is these steps to enlightenment that gives us satisfaction and fulfillment.

Force fields or energy patterns have been discovered to be of primary importance on the subatomic level. The space between subatomic particles is seen to be in many ways the essence of all that occurs. For it is the interaction of the energy and forces that give motion and therefore life to everything we experience with the five senses.

Electric fields affect and can be felt by charged bodies that are separated by distance. Yet they interact and connect through these electric force fields. According to Einstein, the electromagnetic fields of energy, not only connect physical matter but they are the essence of matter itself. He also determined that matter and space are inseparable and interdependent parts of the same whole. These quantum fields of energy are everywhere present in space. Particles of energy and therefore matter are local condensations of this field.

This means the universe is alive in motion, and that what you do through energy interaction affects the rest of the universe. Your thoughts have energy and therefore affect and influence the energy of the rest of the universe. It also indicates what Metaphysicians have always taught: that thoughts are things. It is by your thought of today that you create tomorrow. Thus modern physics justifies and supports the glossary on attitude-diseases. Modern physics has not yet gotten as specific as this list but it is coming in the future.

Electro-magnetic fields are felt physically only by charged bodies which experience their attractive and repulsive forces. However, gravitation fields which are created by all massive bodies such as planets are always attractive. Thus anytime our space program seeks to lift a rocket into space, it takes a tremendous amount of rocket fuel firing (energy) to overcome this attraction of gravity. Gravity becomes a type of entrapment.

Our physical experience is one of entrapment. We are entrapped or engrossed in a physical body. We enter that body at the time of birth and we are trapped in that vehicle until the time of death. During our lifetime, the attractive force of the senses keeps us engrossed for we, being dependent on our senses for experiencing and learning in that environment, begin to believe that the total reality is what we experience with the senses. Thus, we forget that we are a soul or spirit or subconscious mind only inhabiting the body for a lifetime. As we pursue concentration, meditation, and dream interpretation, we begin to experience these higher levels of reality.

A massive body will curve space around itself due to gravitation pull. The gravitational field *is* curved space. People of great attractive charisma or wisdom attract those in their environment to their teaching. Thus space molds itself and forms itself around great individuals due to the powerful creative power of the thoughts, understanding, and knowledge.

In modern physics, there is no place for both the quantum energy field and physical matter, for the energy field is the only reality. So physics has come full turn from describing reality as a dead machine and physical matter as the only reality to one of recognizing the universe as living, energy in motion where reality is made up of condensations of this energy.

And what causes these condensations of energy? The answer is *thoughts*. And what or who produces these thoughts? The answer is consciousness or in other words *you*, a living, breathing, entity. Your thoughts affect and control your world around you and this world around you includes your physical body which is the most immediate environment or vehicle for you the thinker, the soul.

Remember, the illusion of the solid material-physical reality is created by moving particles. Therefore control your own motion by moving forward, rapidly in your life, learning growth and awareness and you control motion. In this fashion the enlightened are fulfilled.

The factors describing the forces between elementary particles are attraction, repulsion, interaction, communication, interdependence, and condensation. The physical exists due to condensation of thought substance from the inner levels of the subconscious and superconscious minds. These condensations first appear as a disturbance of the perfect state of the quantum field. These disturbances are the appearance in the physical of what has already begun in the inner levels of mind. When these subatomic particles disappear out of existence into the void they have actually returned to the inner levels of consciousness from where they came as has always been taught by Metaphysicists. Any thought or desire when created in the conscious mind is transferred to the inner or subconscious mind by the quantum field. Then the thought, through the attractive force, gathers thought or mind substance around it. As the condensation occurs the substance gains enough energy and motion to affect the quantum field and then springs into physical existence. The quantum field is the reality because it is the mediator between what is physical matter and what is non-physical (subconscious, mind substance).

The quantum field being a continuum everywhere present provides the perfect vehicle for the transfer of inner level thought substance to the outer, physical particle granular structure of our matter world. Since the quantum force manifests itself as the exchange of photons between particles and these photons are massless and travel at the speed of light, it is seen that photons exist at the borderline or borderland between matter and mind between the outer, conscious, physical level and the inner, subconscious, mental level of mind.

In the subatomic world, there are no forces. Instead these are interactions between particles. In our everyday experience, we interact with our environment consistently. Therefore in order to create your life as you would will it, thought must be focused and directed to productive creative ends so the power of one's thoughts and attitudes mold your life into the form you desire. Force doesn't exist. Therefore trying to force the results you want will never bring you happiness, for force does not exist. Rather it is the pulsating quantum energy fields that exist. What we deem as power to create is actually the collective effect of multiple exchange.

The uncertainty of the exchange of energy which allows for the creation of mesons (a subatomic particle) is the actual transformation of subconscious mind substance to physical matter energy substance at the moment of shift from vertical, inner level time to horizontal, physical, conscious mind time. These mesons are called virtual particles in modern physics because they are virtually or almost physical. That is, they exist on the borderline between the physical and non-physical or inner levels of mind.

A virtual photon, a type of virtual particle, being massless can traverse indefinite distances and can be created with indefinite small amounts of energy thereby making them the perfect vehicle for the transfer of energy from the inner dimensions or levels of mind to our physical reality.

Physicists say that virtual particles come into being in the physical spontaneously out of the void. Metaphysicists recognize the void to be connected to and existing with the inner levels of mind. The spontaneous appearance of virtual particles out of the void is the well taught movement of creative thought forms from the subconscious dimension of mind to the conscious, physical level. It is this spontaneous appearance of thoughts, thought forms and attitudes into physical reality, that appears as disorder and disease in the physical body. For unproductive thoughts disappear into the void or subconscious mind and later appear spontaneously as virtual particles in the physical body. When these particles have become strengthened, dense, or of sufficient quantity, the attitude appears as disorder or as illness in the body as a direct reflection of limited, unproductive thinking.

Remember, particle interactions create structure thus producing the physical world in which we live. Therefore, the entire universe is one of continual motion and activity. Creation of matter occurs when a photon whose mass is zero and travels at the speed of light, explodes creating an electron and an anti-electron called a positron. Remember also that a photon is a particle of light or in other words a unit of light. Thus matter is seen to be created from light.

Metaphysicists in teaching Self awareness and Self understanding state that at the essence of everyone is light and that the first creation of the creator was light. It was this light differentiating that formed individualized units of light called I AM or individuality as well as the divisions of mind called conscious, subconscious and superconscious.

So creation is built up from:

1) a positive particle, the proton
2) a negative particle, the electron
3) a neutral particle, the neutron
4) a massless particle of light traveling at the speed of Light.

The formula for creation therefore may be stated thus:

proton (+) + *electron* (-) + *neutron* (n) + *photon* (c) = *matter*

This indicates that matter is equal to or made up of positive energy (+), negative energy (-), and a neutral charge (n) activated by the constant speed of Light (c). Thus the speed of Light is seen to be the ultimate limitation of the physical. Our universe is seen to be productive from the aggressive (+) and receptive (-) factors of creation together with a neutral binder that enables them to work together, moderated by the speed of Light.

Of the four particles, the only one that can disintegrate spontaneously is the neutron. This is called beta decay and is a type of radioactivity. Without a neutron, physical matter as we know it does not exist. Radioactivity is a type of rapid breakdown of physical structure. This reminds one of cancer which creates a rapid breakdown of structure in the physical body. It is interesting to note one of the treatments for cancer is radioactive therapy.

Metaphysics teaches it is light using the aggressive and receptive principles through the neutral medium of the mind that creates life and the physical environment. In the subatomic world all particles of a given kind are completely identical. One electron is always identical to another electron. One proton is always identical to another proton.

The mind: conscious, subconscious, and superconscious is constructed according to a definite structure and form based upon the interaction of its constituent parts. In the descent into the subatomic realm we can no longer find ultimate building blocks. When a proton is broken up it forms completely new particles. Therefore, the subatomic structure is a dynamic pattern of change. Since the subatomic forms the foundation for the physical, this means that change is the nature of the physical.

Modern physics states that the manner in which we look at the world determines our physical structural world. Metaphysicists state that we create our world around us with our thoughts and actions. It is our level of awareness that determines the world we live in and create around us. Particles are processes rather than objects. This means our physical reality is one of processes and interactions. These interactions are connected with all other interactions and processes, making for an interconnected universe. Metaphysicists recognize the process is more important than the material object. The action and activity of learning is of utmost importance. The goal or ideal is important to give us direction and the activity provides us with motion to move toward the goal, but it is the purpose which provides the learning from the process and ultimately aids us in our motion towards enlightenment.

The discoveries of modern physics and the awareness of the Metaphysicists are seen to be alike. It is necessary to apply and practice the learning that we create in order to make it a permanent part of ourselves. The observer affects the observed. The experimenter's thoughts affect the experiment. Life is an experiment and we affect the experiment of life. We create and we make a difference therefore each individual is important and has value or worth.

In subatomic physics, particles may communicate with each other at the speed of light or less. However, non-local or faster than light connections have emerged that reflect the interconnectedness of the universe reflected in quantum theory. On the subatomic level non-local connections and communication occurs faster than the speed of light. This is due to the movement from the physical, conscious mind to the inner levels or dimensions of the subconscious mind where time is measured vertically not horizontally. In the end it is seen that the speed of thought breaks or goes beyond the ultimate limitation of the physical, the speed of light.

In physics, an experiment proved Bell's theorem which theorized non-local (faster than the speed of light) connections. The experiment showed that by choosing and measuring the axis of rotation of an electron and by observing an identical particle thousands of miles away, the twin will acquire a different spin as a result. There is instant communication (faster than the speed of light) from one electron to another. It seems that on the level of subatomic particles that the thoughts of the experimenter-observer affect particles over immense distances at faster than the speed of light velocities.

Bell's theorem physically proves a metaphysical truth: thoughts are things and have reality. It also proves that thought directed by intelligence is the most powerful energy in the universe.

The quality of unfoldment in the cosmic web at a deeper unmanifest level is a scientific way of saying it is our duty and purpose to learn and grow, to utilize the universe to gain the experiences necessary to become enlightened. The new scientific world view agrees with Metaphysics - the perennial philosophy.

l) Metaphysics maintains that all people have value and everything one person does affects the rest of the universe. Your relationship to the whole is important and as you aid others in their learning and growth you add also to your own enlightenment.

2) Metaphysics maintains that learning through activity, progressing, reasoning, and building intuition and enlightenment is the process that creates any physical structure.

3) Metaphysics maintains that the individual affects his environment and every experiment he is involved in is affected by him. In fact, life is one large experiment and we the experimenters learn and grow by affecting the environment.

4) Metaphysics maintains that people give value to our lives. To become enlightened one needs others to interact with, to give to, to receive from, to teach, share, and learn from. Relationships are a way to understand ourselves.

5) Metaphysics maintains that not only do thoughts affect reality but thoughts are reality! One's duty is to teach others the universal truths one has discovered. It is only through passing on the learning that we find enlightenment.

6) Through aiding others mankind progresses and we all benefit.

May we all progress together.

Latest Discoveries in Physics Agree with Age Old Metaphysics

Superstring theory, one of the most promising developments of modern physics, posits that all physical phenomena, including the entire physical universe we experience, arise from and are built up from infinitesimal wriggling strings in 10 dimensions.

Metaphysicists have maintained and taught individuals about seven levels of mind for thousands of years. I personally have taught this for over fifteen years. In addition, Metaphysicists have taught and maintained that the "number" of the physical existence is four which represents stability. This is used in a similar manner to notation used in physics such as $E=mc^2$ where "E" symbolizes energy. Four is the number or symbol of the physical because four represents stability.

Physicists, such as Einstein, often use thought-experiements to explain their ideas. Consider this thought experiment: think of a man sitting on a chair. Notice how stable the chair is. Next, imagine a person sitting on a two-legged chair. You will notice this is not as stable, neither is a one-legged or a three-legged chair. A five-legged chair is stable but the fifth leg is not needed and nature tends to do things as efficiently as possible.

The four physical dimensions of nature: length, width, depth, and time, create and form the physical universe around us. The quality of stability is created due to the other six dimensions or levels of mind in the unseen universe. Tetrahedrons, sometimes inaccurately called three-sided pyramids are a solid way or method of explaining ten dimensions. A tetrahedron has four surfaces and six lines. The four surfaces represent the four dimensional solidity of the physical. The six lines represent the subatomic, unseen, or inner levels of mind. The dimension of superstrings.

May permanent healing be yours.

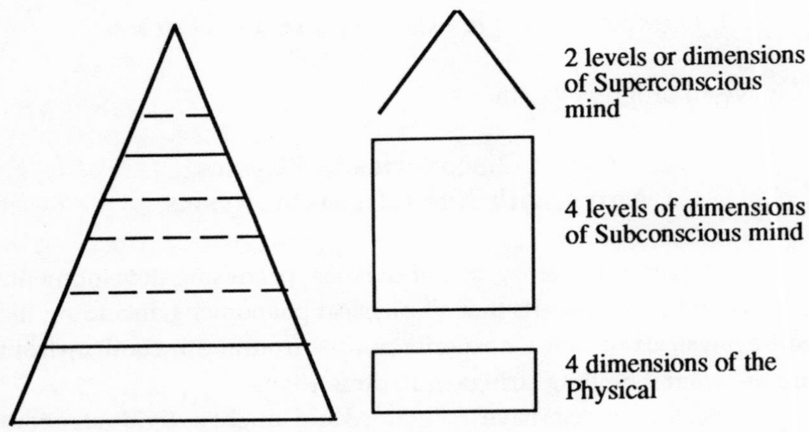

Geometric Diagram
of 10 dimensions of mind

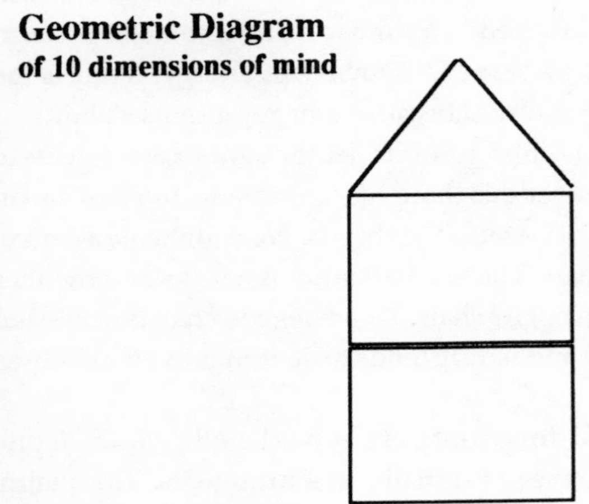

About the Author

Daniel R. Condron, D.M., D.D., M.S., Ps.D., was born in Chillicothe, Missouri. Raised on a farm ten miles from that town, he excelled in sports and academics during his high school years. Condron furthered his education at the University of Missouri - Columbia where he earned Bachelors and Masters degrees. He traveled throughout Europe and South America, and was named to Who's Who in American Colleges and Universities. Condron has devoted the last thirty years of his life to Self awareness and understanding the universal language of mind.

In addition to being known as an author, Condron is well respected as a teacher, lecturer, counselor, poet, and sales and management consultant. An international lecturer, he is often the keynote or featured speaker at seminars and universities throughout the country. Serving as a teacher of mind and spirit to people throughout the country, Condron is President of the Board of Directors of the School of Metaphysics, an educational and service institute with centers throughout the Midwest and headquartered in Missouri. His influence continues to reach around the globe as a conductor of readings, including the Health Analyses, offered through the institute.

Condron looks forward to aiding millions of people to lead a richer and more rewarding life.

Additional titles available from SOM Publishing include:

Dreams of the Soul - The Yogi Sutras of Patanjali
Dr. Daniel R. Condron ISBN 0944386-11-3 $9.95

Meditation: Answer to Your Prayers by Dr. Jerry L. Rothermel
ISBN 0944386-01-6 $4.95

Going in Circles - Search for a Satisfying Relationship
Dr. Barbara G. Rothermel ISBN 0944386-00-8 $5.95

What Will I Do Tomorrow? Probing Depression
Dr. Barbara G. Rothermel ISBN 0944386-02-4 $4.95

Who Were Those Strangers in My Dream?
Dr. Barbara G. Rothermel ISBN 0944386-08-3 $4.95

Dreams: Language of the Soul by Dr. Jerry L. Rothermel
ISBN 0944386-04-0 $4.95

Symbols of Dreams by Dr. Jerry L. Rothermel
ISBN 0944386-03-2 $4.95

Mechanics of Dreams by Dr. Jerry L. Rothermel
ISBN 0944386-09-1 $6.95

Discovering the Kingdom of Heaven by Dr. Gayle B. Matthes
ISBN 0944386-07-5 $5.95

Autobiography of a Skeptic by Frank Farmer
ISBN 0944386-06-7 $7.95

HuMan, a novel by Dr. Jerry L. Rothermel
ISBN 0944386-05-9 $5.95

to be released in 1992....

Beyond Phenomena - Readings from the Akasha
edited by Dr. Barbara O'Guinn ISBN 0944386-10-5 $9.95

Kundalini Rising - Mastering Your Creative Energies
Dr. Barbara O'Guinn ISBN 0944386-13-X $9.95

To order, or for a catalogue of all titles available, write:

SOM Publishing
School of Metaphysics
National Headquarters
Windyville, Missouri 65783

Enclose a check or money order payable to SOM with any order. Please include $2.00 for postage and handling of books.